RNA Therapeutics - History, Design, Manufacturing, and Applications

Edited by Irina Vlasova-St. Louis

Published in London, United Kingdom

RNA Therapeutics - History, Design, Manufacturing, and Applications
http://dx.doi.org/10.5772/intechopen.102166
Edited by Irina Vlasova-St. Louis

Contributors
Akihide Yoshimi, Michiko Kurikawa, Marimu Sakumoto, Hock Siew Tan, Bao Chi Wong, Umama Shahid, Manish K. Tripathi, Ana Ayala Pazzi, Puneet Vij, Nura Salhadar, Elias George, Irina Vlasova-St. Louis, Jude Abadie, Clévio Nóbrega, José Codêsso, Carlos A. Matos

First published in London, United Kingdom, 2023 by IntechOpen
IntechOpen is the global imprint of INTECHOPEN LIMITED, registered in England and Wales, registration number: 11086078, 5 Princes Gate Court, London, SW7 2QJ, United Kingdom

British Library Cataloguing-in-Publication Data
A catalogue record for this book is available from the British Library

Additional hard and PDF copies can be obtained from orders@intechopen.com

RNA Therapeutics - History, Design, Manufacturing, and Applications
Edited by Irina Vlasova-St. Louis
p. cm.
Print ISBN 978-1-80355-657-4
Online ISBN 978-1-80355-658-1
eBook (PDF) ISBN 978-1-80355-659-8

Meet the editor

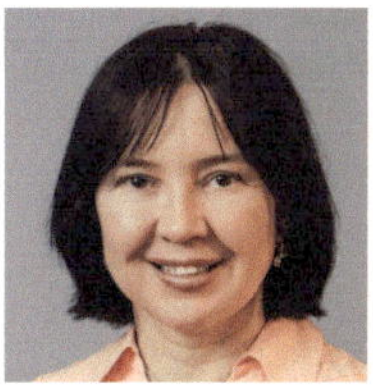

Dr. Irina Vlasova-St. Louis obtained her MD and Ph.D. from Ural State Medical Academy, Russia. She completed her post-doctoral training at the University of Minnesota, USA, and a laboratory fellowship sponsored by the Lymphoma Research Foundation. She served as an assistant professor at the University of Minnesota, Department of Medicine, providing expertise in several biological disciplines including infectious diseases, immunology, genomics, and bioinformatics. During the COVID-19 pandemic, Dr. Vlasova-St. Louis led genomic surveillance of circulating SARS-CoV-2 variants of concern in Nevada, USA. Currently, she is a genomics specialist at the Newborn Screening Department, Texas Department of State Health Services, USA. She is sponsored by federal grants from the Association of Public Health Laboratories and Centers for Disease Control and Prevention. She is a part of the Johns Hopkins University Advanced Academic Program: Individualized Genomics and Health.

Contents

Preface **IX**

Section 1
Introduction **1**

Chapter 1 **3**
Introductory Chapter: RNA Drugs Development and Commercialization
by Irina Vlasova-St. Louis

Section 2
RNA Vaccines and Drugs against Infectious Diseases **11**

Chapter 2 **13**
Prophylactic Ribonucleic Acid Vaccines to Combat RNA Viral Infections in Humans
by Irina Vlasova-St. Louis and Jude Abadie

Chapter 3 **37**
Ribozymes as Therapeutic Agents against Infectious Diseases
by Bao Chi Wong, Umama Shahid and Hock Siew Tan

Section 3
Anti-Cancer RNA Therapeutics **61**

Chapter 4 **63**
A New Era of RNA Personalized Vaccines for Cancer and Cancer-Causing Infectious Diseases
by Ana Ayala Pazzi, Puneet Vij, Nura Salhadar, Elias George and Manish K. Tripathi

Chapter 5 **79**
Perspective Chapter: RNA Therapeutics for Cancers
by Michiko Kurikawa, Marimu Sakumoto and Akihide Yoshimi

Section 4
RNA Drugs for Rare Diseases **103**

Chapter 6 **105**
RNA Interference Applications for Machado-Joseph Disease
by José M. Codêsso, Carlos A. Matos and Clévio Nóbrega

Preface

"It's time for scientists to shout about RNA therapies"
Lorna Harries (Nature 574, S15. 2019)

RNA Therapeutics - History, Design, Manufacturing, and Applications addresses recent advances in RNA-based drug discovery and commercialization. The design and development of RNA drugs have resulted in several distinct classes of treatment known as nucleic acid therapies. Chapter 1: "Introductory Chapter: RNA Drugs Development and Commercialization" describes and discusses these therapies, which include an impressive list of mRNA, SARNA, miRNA, siRNA, RNA analogs, ribozymes, antisense oligonucleotides, and CRISPR-based drugs.

The COVID-19 pandemic spurred a burst of development of mRNA vaccines, which culminated in rapid mRNA vaccine testing and approval for use in humans. Chapter 2 "Prophylactic Ribonucleic Acid Vaccines to Combat RNA Viral Infections in Humans" discusses these vaccines, while Chapter 3 "Ribozymes as Therapeutic Agents against Infectious Diseases" discusses therapeutic ribozymes.

Applications of RNA therapeutics range from infectious disease prophylaxis to treating cancer and chronic conditions, improving organ transplant outcomes, and correcting inherited mutations. Chapter 4: "A New Era of RNA Personalized Vaccines for Cancer and Cancer-Causing Infectious Diseases" discusses RNA therapeutics for various types of malignancies originatingfrom chronic viral infections or somatic mutations. Chapter 5: "Perspective Chapter: RNA Therapeutics for Cancers" reviews distinct classes of RNA therapeutics as well as examines the challenges in RNA drug engineering, delivery, and improvement of pharmacological effectiveness.

The optimization of RNA-based therapeutics enables countless opportunities in our pursuit of achieving the goals of individualized medicine. This is particularly applicable to rare genetic disorders for which RNA drugs may provide a cure. As such, Chapter 6: "RNA Interference Applications for Machado-Joseph Disease" discusses applications of RNA interferences for a rare neurodegenerative disease caused by abnormal expansion of trinucleotide repeats in non-coding regions of RNAs.

RNA therapeutics have significantly impacted medicine, economy, and overall public health and thus hold great promise to modernize health care.

Irina Vlasova-St. Louis, MD, Ph.D.
Individualized Genomics and Health Program,
Johns Hopkins University,
Baltimore, MD, USA

Genomics Specialist,
Molecular Branch of Newborn Screening Program,
Texas Department of State Health Services,
Austin, Texas, USA

Section 1

Introduction

Chapter 1

Introductory Chapter: RNA Drugs Development and Commercialization

Irina Vlasova-St. Louis

1. Introduction

RNA therapeutics are chemically synthesized biomolecules with broad clinical applications, ranging from correcting inherited mutations to treating cancer, chronic conditions, improving organ transplant outcomes, and infectious disease prophylaxes (**Figure 1**).

2. Applications of RNA-based therapeutics in medicine

The development of RNA therapeutics has been an intense journey, with numerous stories of success and failure. The potential, and suitability, of recently discovered RNAs stemmed from several Nobel Prize-winning discoveries. For example, the Nobel prize for messenger RNA discovery was awarded to F. Jacob, J. Monod, and A. Lwoff in 1965 [1]. Almost 30 years later, P. Sharp and R. Roberts were presented with the Nobel Prize for the discovery of alternative mRNA splicing. The idea for mRNA

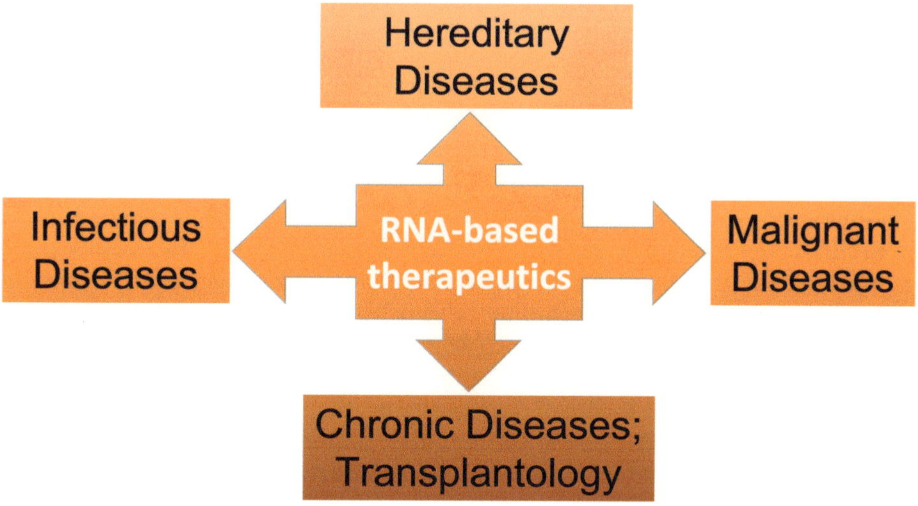

Figure 1.
Applications of RNA-based therapeutics in medicine that are discussed in this book.

technologies as biopharmaceuticals for infectious and oncological diseases materialized in the early twenty-first century. Two companies, BioNTech and Moderna, which were founded two years apart (in 2008 and 2010, respectively), began working on the commercialization of mRNA-based vaccines against flu and subsequently Ebola disease [2]. The COVID-19 pandemic has speeded up mRNA technologies and culminated in rapid mRNA vaccine testing and approval for use in humans. RNA-based therapeutic vaccines (e.g., those developed to fight against SARS-CoV-2 infection) have been proven to be safe and effective. Several of the vaccines were approved by the FDA and the European Commission (EC).

An interesting formulation of double-stranded RNAs is one which activates TLR-3 receptors. This drug is sold under the generic name Rintatolimod in South America and Canada. The drug is indicated for treatment of patients with chronic fatigue syndrome, a poorly understood complication of many viral infections [3]. RNA drugs have great therapeutic potential to modulate inflammatory responses and combat oxidative stress to prevent tissue and organ damage during severe infections; however, the investigations of RNA drug utility are still at the pre-clinical stage [4, 5]. Greater attention has been devoted to antiviral RNA therapeutics, several of which have progressed to clinical phases 2 and 3, including Favipiravir (against Ebola Disease) and siRNA drugs for the treatment of chronic hepatitis B and HPV virus infections [6–8]. The anti-SARS-CoV-2 RNA analogs Ledipasvir and Remdesivir have recently been granted FDA approval to treat COVID-19 infection [9–11].

RNA therapies are evolving as individualized treatment solutions for cancer. In 2006, Nobel Prize was shared by Professors A. Fire and C. Mello for their discovery of gene silencing by double-stranded RNA interference (RNAi) [1]. siRNAs (as well as miRNAs) have been tested to inhibit overexpressed genes in various malignant tumors, including multiple myeloma, pancreatic, and hepatocellular carcinomas [12]. Unfortunately, the side effects that were observed in the studies' participants along with poor efficacy resulted in the termination of many studies.

Antisense Oligonucleotides (ASO) became the number one choice for therapeutic design in the early twenty-first century to treat cancers that resulted from oncogene duplication or overexpression (e.g., C-MYB, BCL, IGF1R) [13]. Several ASO therapeutics have been incorporated into the conventional treatment of oncological diseases, including chronic lymphocytic leukemia (CLL), diffuse large B-cell lymphoma (DLBCL), and glioblastoma [14]. More recently, RNA aptamers and raptamers have been tested as multifunctional RNA drugs in the field of oncology [15]. For example, bi-specific aptamers were designed to activate receptors on tumor-infiltrating T cells against cancer-associated receptors. The aptamers linked to a siRNA against the gene of interest can downregulate the target gene directly in tumor cells or modulate tumor cell immunogenicity, thus enhancing anti-tumor immune response. Aptamers conjugated to chemotherapeutic molecules can be delivered in a cell-specific manner (e.g., if designed to bind tumor oncomarkers) [15]. Such properties significantly expand the portfolio of malignant diseases, including cancers with immunosuppressive properties.

Human trials of non-formulated mRNA- and mRNA-based dendritic-cell cancer vaccines have been taking place since the mid-2000s. Several dozens of ongoing clinical trials are well described in [16]. The majority of them is designed as study arms in combination with standard immune checkpoint therapies or individualized biologics to treat devastating cancers such as glioma, melanoma, prostate cancer, and non-small-cell lung, pancreatic, and colorectal neoplasms. The future goal is to achieve targeted delivery, attune kinetics of mRNA expression, overcome cancer mutation rate, and reduce unintended host-immune reactions [17].

siRNA drugs has become invaluable in the field of transplantology, where life-saving hematopoietic stem cell transplantation is accompanied by numerous pre- and post-transplant complications [18, 19]. One of the complications is hepatic veno-occlusive disease/sinusoidal obstructive syndrome (VOD/SOS), which has been successfully treated by the drug Defibrotide, which was formulated as a mixture of single- and double-stranded oligonucleotides [20]. Patients who undergo transplantation procedures are often at high risk for GVHD and acute kidney injury, which now can be mitigated by siRNA against p53 mRNA (Teprasiran, Quark-Pharmaceuticals) [21].

Alnylam, a U.S.-based company, is pioneering siRNA treatments against rare hereditary diseases. Several siRNA drugs have already been approved by the FDA and granted orphan drug designation [22]:

- Vutrisiran and Patisiran target TTR in patients with hereditary variant transthyretin amyloidosis and hereditary TTR-mediated polyneuropathy/cardiomyopathy [23, 24];

- Inclisiran was designed to knockdown PCSK9 in patients with homozygous familial hypercholesterolemia [25];

- Lumasiran and Nedosiran were designed to knockdown HAO1 and LDHA genes, respectively, to treat primary hyperoxalurias type I–III [26, 27];

- Givosiran is a siRNA drug that targets the ALAS1 gene as a treatment for acute hepatic porphyria (AHP) [28].

Another group of rare diseases, hemophilia A and hemophilia B, are being evaluated for management with monthly subcutaneous administration of siRNA-based therapy fitusiran (Sanofi) [29]. Currently, novel siRNA drugs are entering clinical trials almost daily; information about them can be found at clinicaltrials.gov and ema.europa.eu/en/medicines. Many pre-clinical studies are in progress at academic institutions and biopharmaceutical companies [30].

S. Altman and T. Cech were awarded a Nobel prize for the discovery of catalytic RNAs, now named Ribozymes [1]. This diverse group of single-stranded RNAs acts as enzymes when folded into secondary and tertiary structures [31]. Several clinical trials investigated the utility of Ribozymes in the treatment of HIV-infected individuals [32, 33]. Therapeutic Ribozymes were designed and tested against angiogenic factor VEGF1, which is often overexpressed in cancer; however, due to higher interest in the commercialization of RNAi-based therapies, Ribozyme trials eventually stopped.

E. Charpentier and J. Doudna received the Nobel Price for the discovery of CRISPR-Cas in the middle of the COVID-19 pandemic [34]. CRISPR technology, which was initially designed to disrupt the gene of interest for experimentation, now is thought to be applied to treat inherited diseases. CRISPR-Cas is becoming a great alternative to siRNA therapeutic applications [35].

There are estimated 5000–8000 rare monogenic diseases that can be cured by gene therapies, including CRISPR-Cas [36]. Commercialization of CRISPR technology leads to several clinical trials that utilize CRISPR-Cas9 modalities to correct mutations that cause sickle cell anemia, β-thalassemia, cystic fibrosis, Duchenne muscular dystrophy, Huntington's chorea, and hereditary retinal degenerative diseases [24, 37]. The versatility of CRISPR-Cas therapeutic applications is wide and has the potential to provide twenty-first-century cures to newborns. Additionally, it may even provide cures, preconceptionally, to families affected by the genetic disease.

3. Conclusions

This book presents distinct classes of RNA therapeutics, ranging from single-stranded antisense oligonucleotides (ASOs) and subclasses of RNA interferences (miRNAs and other RNAi) to *in vitro* transcribed mRNAs and RNA vaccines. Also presented are some of the challenges in RNA drug engineering, delivery, and specificity. Additionally, the improvement of pharmacological effectiveness is discussed.

RNA therapeutics have already had a significant impact on medicine, the economy, and overall public health. They are becoming prescription drugs, and this holds great promise for modernizing healthcare [38]. National Genome Research Institute has recently launched a genotype-first approach to trace genomic variants back to human disorders. Accumulated data on human genome sequencing may inevitably lead us to a preventive medicine mindset. Monumental breakthroughs in molecular biology, computational chemistry, bioinformatics, and individualized genomics, which undoubtedly propelled RNA therapeutics through the commercialization stage, are also examined in this book.

Acknowledgements

I am thankful for the grant support received from the Association of Public Health Laboratories (APHL) during the editing of this book.

Conflict of interest

None declared.

Acronyms and abbreviations

FDA	United States Food and Drug Administration
EC	European Commission
TLR-3	toll-like receptor
CRISPR	clustered regularly interspaced short palindromic repeats
IGF-1R	IGF type-1 receptor
miRNA	micro RNA
siRNA	small interfering RNA
CRISPR/Cas	clustered regularly interspaced short palindromic repeats/ CRISPR-associated
PCSK9	proprotein convertase subtilisin kexin type 9
TTR	transthyretin gene
PH	primary hyperoxaluria
LDH	lactate dehydrogenase
ALAS1	aminolevulinic acid synthase
AHP	acute hepatic porphyria
GVHD	graft versus host disease

Author details

Irina Vlasova-St. Louis[1,2]

1 Individualized Genomics and Health Program, Johns Hopkins University, Baltimore, MD, USA

2 Molecular Branch of Newborn Screening Program, Texas Department of State Health Services, Austin, Texas, USA

*Address all correspondence to: stlouis.irina@gmail.com; istloui1@alumni.jh.edu

References

[1] The Nobel Prize. Nobel Prize Laureates. Available from: https://www.nobelprize.org/ [Accessed: December 26, 2022]

[2] Vlasova-St. Louis I, Abadie J. Prophylactic ribonucleic acid vaccines to combat rna viral infections in humans. In: RNA Therapeutics - History, Design, Manufacturing, and Applications. London, UK: IntechOpen; 2022. pp. 14-38

[3] AIM ImmunoTech. As Rintatolimod Moves Closer to Clinical Approval, What is the Likelihood that the Drug will be Approved?. Available from: https://www.pharmaceutical-technology.com/data-analysis/rintatolimod-what-is-the-likelihood-that-drug-will-be-approved/ [Accessed: December 30, 2022]

[4] Martínez T, Jiménez AI, Pañeda C. Short-interference RNAs: Becoming medicines. EXCLI Journal. 2015;**14**:714-176

[5] Veiga N, Goldsmith M, Diesendruck Y, et al. Leukocyte-specific siRNA delivery revealing IRF8 as a potential anti-inflammatory target. Journal of Controlled Release. 2019;**313**:33-41

[6] Flisiak R, Jaroszewicz J, Łucejko M. siRNA drug development against hepatitis B virus infection. Expert Opinion on Biological Therapy. 2018;**18**:609-617

[7] ClinicalTrials.gov. A Study Evaluating Treatment Regimens Containing Vebicorvir (ABI-H0731) in Participants With Chronic Hepatitis B Infection. 2021. NCT04820686. Available from: https://clinicaltrials.gov/ct2/show/NCT04820686

[8] ClinicalTrials.gov. Primary Organoid Models and Combined Nucleic Acids Therapeutics for Anti-HPV Treatments (ORGANOIDES). Available from: https://clinicaltrials.gov/ct2/show/NCT04278326 [Accessed: January 01, 2023]

[9] Aschenbrenner DS. Remdesivir approved to treat COVID-19 amid controversy. American Journal of Nursing. 2021;**121**:22-24

[10] Agrawal U, Raju R, Udwadia ZF. Favipiravir: A new and emerging antiviral option in COVID-19. Medical Journal, Armed Forces India. 2020;**76**:370-376

[11] Jose M, Kuttchira P. Current therapeutic options for Coronoviruses disease-2019—A pharmacological review. Asian Journal of Pharmaceutical and Clinical Research. 2020;**13**:42-50

[12] Feng R, Patil S, Zhao X, et al. RNA therapeutics—Research and clinical advancements. Frontiers in Molecular Biosciences. 2021;**8**:1-7

[13] Jiang C, Meng L, Yang B, et al. Application of CRISPR/Cas9 gene editing technique in the study of cancer treatment. Clinical Genetics. 2020;**97**:73-88

[14] Kurikawa M, Sakumoto M, Yoshimi A. RNA therapeutics for cancers. In: RNA Therapeutics - History, Design, Manufacturing, and Applications. London, UK: IntechOpen; 2022. pp. 1-24

[15] Shigdar S, Schrand B, Giangrande PH, et al. Aptamers: Cutting edge of cancer therapies. Molecular Therapy. 2021;**29**:2396-2411

[16] Lorentzen C, Haanen J, Met Ö, et al. Clinical advances and ongoing trials of mRNA vaccines for cancer treatment. The Lancet Oncology. 2022;**23**:E450-E458

[17] Miao L, Zhang Y, Huang L. mRNA vaccine for cancer immunotherapy. Molecular Cancer. 2021;**20**:41-44

[18] Kellampalli U, Mohei H, Vlasova-St. Louis I. Kinetics of immune reconstitution and immune complications after cell and organ transplantation. Integrative Cancer Science and Therapeutics. 2020;7:2-6

[19] Bejanyan N, Vlasova-St Louis I, Mohei H, et al. Cytomegalovirus-specific immunity recovers more slowly after cord blood transplantation compared with matched sibling donor allogeneic transplantation. Transplantation and Cellular Therapy. 2021;**27**(187):e1-e4

[20] Nauffal M, Kim HT, Richardson PG, et al. Defibrotide: Real-world management of veno-occlusive disease/sinusoidal obstructive syndrome after stem cell transplant. Blood Advance. 2022;**6**:181-188

[21] ClinicalTrials.gov. QPI-1002 for Prevention of Delayed Graft Function in Recipients of an Older Donor Kidney Transplant (ReGIFT). Available from: https://clinicaltrials.gov/ct2/show/NCT02610296 [Accessed: January 01, 2023]

[22] Friedrich M, Aigner A. Therapeutic siRNA: State-of-the-art and future perspectives. BioDrugs. 2022;**36**:549-571

[23] Adams D, Tournev I, Taylor M, et al. HELIOS-A: 9-month results from the phase 3 study of vutrisiran in patients with hereditary transthyretin-mediated amyloidosis with polyneuropathy. Journal of Neurological Science. 2021;**429**:117767

[24] Yamashita T, Ueda M, Koike H, et al. Patisiran, an RNAi therapeutic for patients with hereditary transthyretin-mediated amyloidosis: Sub-analysis in Japanese patients from the APOLLO study. Neurology and Clinical Neuroscience. 2020;**8**:251-260

[25] Larkin HD. Injectable siRNA approved for lowering cholesterol. JAMA. 2022;**327**:805

[26] Hulton SA. Lumasiran: Expanding the treatment options for patients with primary hyperoxaluria type 1. Expert Opinion on Orphan Drugs. 2021;**9**:189-198

[27] Liu A, Zhao J, Shah M, et al. Nedosiran, a candidate siRNA drug for the treatment of primary Hyperoxaluria: Design, development, and clinical studies. ACS Pharmacology and Translational Science. 2022;**2022**:1007-1016

[28] grugbank.com. Givosiran. Available from: https://go.drugbank.com/drugs/DB15066 [Accessed: January 01, 2023]

[29] Sanofi. Press Release: Fitusiran Prophylaxis Reduced Bleeds by 61% in People with Hemophilia A or B, with or without Inhibitors, Compared to Prior Factor or Bypassing Agent Prophylaxis. Available from: https://www.sanofi.com/en/media-room/press-releases/2022/2022-07-10-13-45-00-2476896 [Accessed: January 01, 2023]

[30] Codêsso JM, Matos CA, Nóbrega C. RNA interference applications for Machado-Joseph disease. In: RNA Therapeutics - History, Design, Manufacturing, and Applications. London, UK: IntechOpen; 2022. pp. 1-23

[31] Wong BC, Shahid U, Tan HS. Ribozymes as therapeutic agents against infectious diseases. In: RNA Therapeutics - History, Design, Manufacturing, and Applications. London, UK: IntechOpen; 2022. pp. 1-23

[32] Mitsuyasu RT, Merigan TC, Carr A, et al. Phase 2 gene therapy trial of an

anti-HIV ribozyme in autologous CD34 + cells. Nature Medicine. 2009;**15**:258-292

[33] Vishnu P, Aboulafia DM. AIDS-related non-hodgkin's lymphoma in the era of highly active antiretroviral therapy. Advances in Hematology. 2012;**2012**:1-9

[34] Westermann L, Neubauer B, Köttgen M. Nobel prize 2020 in chemistry honors CRISPR: A tool for rewriting the code of life. Pflugers Archiv: European Journal of Physiology. 2021;**473**:1-2

[35] Jiang L, Wang LY, Cheng XS. Novel approaches for the treatment of familial hypercholesterolemia: Current status and future challenges. Journal of Atherosclerosis and Thrombosis. 2018;**25**:665-673

[36] Condò I. Rare monogenic diseases: Molecular pathophysiology and novel therapies. International Journal of Molecular Science. 2022;**23**:6525-6529

[37] ClinicalTrials.gov. Single Ascending Dose Study in Participants with LCA10. Available from: https://clinicaltrials.gov/ct2/show/NCT03872479 [Accessed: January 01, 2023]

[38] Arabi F, Mansouri V, Ahmadbeigi N. Gene therapy clinical trials, where do we go? An overview. Biomedicine and Pharmacotherapy. 2022;**153**:113324

Section 2

RNA Vaccines and Drugs against Infectious Diseases

Chapter 2

Prophylactic Ribonucleic Acid Vaccines to Combat RNA Viral Infections in Humans

Irina Vlasova-St. Louis and Jude Abadie

Abstract

Vaccines have evolved as widely applicable and available prophylaxes against infectious diseases. Advances in ribonucleic acid technologies revolutionized the biopharmaceutical field of vaccine manufacturing. Numerous novel mRNA-based vaccines that have been approved by the United States and European regulatory agencies are proven to be safe and effective in preventing disease. This chapter presents the history of RNA vaccine development in the context of preventing diseases caused by RNA viruses such as SARS-CoV-2, HIV, influenza, Chikungunya, Zika, RSV, PIV, HMPV viruses, Rabies, and Ebola. Advantages, disadvantages, and challenges in mRNA vaccine engineering, delivery, and safety are discussed. The formulation, safety, long-term effectiveness, and requirements for booster immunizations are presented using data from clinical trials. The results of these clinical trials highlight important milestones, setbacks, and ultimate advancements in vaccine development. mRNA vaccines have significantly impacted public health in a relatively short time, and they demonstrate great potential in serving as clinical public health prophylaxis against current and future pandemics. Future development is likely to include polyvalent, mosaic, and strain/lineage-specific individualized vaccines.

Keywords: prophylactic vaccines, mRNA vaccines, SARNA vaccines, RNA viruses, SARS-CoV-2, influenza, HIV, RSV, parainfluenza type 3 virus, human Metapneumovirus, chikungunya, Zika virus, COVID-19, Ebola, epidemic, pandemic, clinical trials, genomics surveillance, public health, emergency preparedness

1. Introduction

The history of vaccines development continually demonstrates their evolution as prophylaxes agents against the spread of disease. For example, as demonstrated with annual flu immunizations, vaccinations have been key in establishing herd immunity and preventing outbreaks of infectious diseases. The pandemic resulting from SARS-CoV-2 infections necessitated vaccine development in a fashion that was accelerated compared to standard regulatory approval processes. Biopharmaceutical companies initiated vaccine research and development as soon as SARS-CoV-2 sequencing data become available. This led to rapid and seamless transitions to clinical trials using conventional vaccine candidates, as well as mRNA vaccines.

Next-generation RNA sequencing continues to evolve as the primary method public health laboratories use to conduct genomic epidemiology surveillance. This is particularly important for novel zoonotic infections that can cross inter-species barriers with the potential to cause epidemics and, perhaps, pandemics. RNA viruses demonstrate continual genetic recombination, in conjunction with the rapid accumulation of mutations, due to the inefficient proofreading ability of viral replicases. Therefore, real-time viral genotyping is of critical importance to public health during outbreaks resulting from virulent RNA viruses. Genotyping data became the fundamental basis for vaccine design. Furthermore, it provided insight into vaccine breakthroughs and allowed vaccine optimization through transgene sequence modifications.

The four types of conventional vaccines include live-attenuated vaccines, whole-pathogen inactivated vaccines, toxoid vaccines, and recombinant protein vaccines [1]. Inactivated vaccines and live-attenuated vaccines contain the whole pathogen. Live-attenuated vaccines (for example, against yellow fever, chickenpox, rotavirus, smallpox, or combined vaccine against measles, mumps, rubella (MMR)), are produced through various attenuation procedures [2]. These vaccines are quite immunogenic, and they can induce long-lasting humoral (systemic or mucosal) and cellular immune responses. However, whole virion vaccines are costly because viruses must be grown in cell cultures during commercial production [3]. There is a risk of reversion of live attenuated vaccines to a wild form, and this is why they are contraindicated for immunocompromised individuals. Poliovirus, hepatitis A, influenza, and rabies are the most successful inactivated vaccines. They can be conveniently freeze-dried for transport; however, large doses of virion administration are required, which can cause unintended adverse events due to host immune reactions. Additionally, the inactivation process may alter immunogenic epitopes confirmation, which makes vaccines less effective [4]. Toxoid vaccines immunize against toxins, which are produced by some bacterial pathogens (e.g., tetanus).

Recombinant DNA technologies produced recombinant protein vaccines. These vaccines were considered safer, with fewer adverse events in clinical trials. However, the identification of the best immunogenic antigen and the complexity of manufacturing design lengthened pre-clinical studies from several years to decades [4]. Protein vaccines often require adjuvants or conjugates to improve immunogenicity, stabilizers to maintain antigen conformation, and other nanomaterials – to improve internalization by antigen-presenting cells (APCs) *in vivo* [4]. The examples of most recent protein vaccines are hepatitis B and human papillomavirus (HPV). Traditionally, the development and production of these conventional vaccine types have been laborious and costly; furthermore, many of them lacked the efficacy to attain post-market approval.

Advances in nucleic acid technologies revolutionized the biopharmaceutical field of vaccine manufacturing. The ability of two novel types of vaccines, mRNA and DNA-based, to produce protein inside the immunized organisms, opened a new era in vaccinology [5]. However, unlike protein vaccines that are formulated without cargo, the DNA and mRNA vaccines required vehicles so that they could be delivered into cells [6]. Upon immunization, DNA vaccines use either plasmid or viral vectors to deliver the transgene into cells. Various lipid nanoparticle cargos have recently been developed for mRNA vaccines to increase the efficiency of cytoplasmic delivery. The poor stability of mRNA molecules (*ex vivo* and in *vivo*) requires additional considerations for formulation and storage (**Table 1**) [7]. Several biochemical solutions for RNA chemistries and lipid nanoparticle design have been proposed and thoroughly reviewed [8–11]. The major challenge identified for mRNA-based vaccines is achieving

Vaccine type	Advantages	Disadvantages
Nonreplicating or non-amplifying mRNA vaccines	Non-viral cytosolic delivery with biodegradable lipo-particles Transient translation of mRNA improves the safety profile Large-scale vaccine production Elicit cell-mediated and humoral immune responses Easy to modify	RNase free conditions is required during manufacturing Low temperature storage is required Host immune response to exogenous mRNA results in inhibition of translation Transient translation might result in low amount of antigen production
Self-replicating or self-amplifying RNA vaccines	Non-viral cytosolic delivery with biodegradable lipo-particles Multiple rounds of replication in the cytoplasm (lower doses are needed) SARNAs are presented by both major histocompatibility complexes 1 and 2 (endogenous adjuvant) Elicit humoral and functional T cell responses against antigen Easy to modify	More complexed manufacturing is required due to two separate RNA formulations Low temperature storage is required Sensitive to RNases Elicit innate host immune response which may inhibit translation
DNA-based vaccines	Good thermostability Fast internalization into cells via fusion mechanism Efficient transcription of the transgene upon nuclear delivery Non-replicative virus design Transient episomal transcription from newer adenoviral vectors	Complexed manufacturing of viral particles Low success of plasmid-based delivery of viral components Risk of host genome integration and promoter-driven expression of host oncogenes Host immune response to the vector upon booster

See text for references.

Table 1.
Advantages and disadvantages of DNA and RNA-based vaccines.

effective *in vivo* translation and identifying the correct/optimal dose of immunogen [12]. Therefore, despite the cost-effectiveness of *in vitro* synthesized mRNA vaccines and the potential for attaining large-scale manufacturing, the formulation of mRNA vaccines for delivery was an obstacle for several decades that has recently been overcome [13]. The history of successes and failures in vaccine development against infections caused by RNA viruses is elucidated throughout the literature review for infections caused by the Ebola virus, SARS-CoV-2, rabies, Zika, HIV, influenza, and the respiratory syncytial virus (RSV).

2. SARS-CoV-2 RNA vaccines

Coronaviruses are enveloped and contain between 25 and 32 Kb of non-segmented positive-sense RNA. Before the emergence of SARS-CoV-2, coronaviruses caused sporadic epidemics around the world [14, 15]. As described in [16], early during the COVID-19 outbreak, next-generation sequencing (NGS) of SARS-CoV-2 RNA provided valuable data about viral genome, its molecular origin, and a deeper understanding of pathogenicity.

As the COVID-19 pandemic spread, the world anxiously anticipated vaccine countermeasures [17]. At that time, mRNA vaccine development was the scientific leader in our fight to end the pandemic. It is nothing short of spectacular heroism and scientific acuity that novel, effective mRNA vaccines were developed in less than 1 year and awarded emergency use authorization (EUA) in the United States. EUA authority allows the Food and Drug Administration (FDA) to approve medical products in order to diagnose, treat, or prevent life-threatening diseases during times or circumstances when no viable alternatives exist during public health emergencies. The Secretary of the US State and Human Services declared the COVID-19 public health emergency on January 31, 2020.

The first batch of Moderna's mRNA-1273 was released for Phase 1 study in the United States in February 2020. This vaccine targeted the receptor binding domain of the Spike protein subunit and was encapsulated in lipid nanoparticles. The cytosolic delivery and temporary presence of mRNA in the cytoplasm improved the safety profile of these nucleic acid vaccines. To assess safety, Pfizer and BioNTech launched phases 1 and 2 clinical trials with the mRNA vaccine during the subsequent months. The primary goal for the phase 2 trial was to achieve *in vivo* protein translation and induction of humoral immune responses upon intramuscular injection. When phases 1 and 2 were successfully completed, the FDA approved phase 3 in conjunction with EUA-authorized vaccine use [18, 19]. While perhaps not expected, it was quickly realized that mRNA vaccines were neither 100% effective nor 100% safe. Subsequent infections, caused by SARS-CoV-2 lineage Omicron, were accompanied by numerous vaccine breakthroughs. Fortunately, novel variants have been associated with milder diseases demonstrated by lower rates of morbidity and mortality. Investigational findings after showed that the anti-SARS-CoV-2 neutralizing antibody titers declined about six months after initial vaccination, which supported recommendations for a booster vaccination. Booster vaccines, like the initial vaccinations, were neither fully effective nor safe. Adverse reactions reported among vaccinations include myocarditis, thyroiditis, systemic vasculitis, and vaccine-associated pulmonary immunopathology [20–22].

Another new type of vaccine known as self-amplifying RNAs (SARNA) has recently completed pre-clinical studies [23]. SARNAs are synthetic RNAs capable of *in vivo* self-amplification for 40 to 60 rounds, a feature supported by their delivery with an alphavirus replicase gene that encodes an RNA-dependent RNA polymerase (RdRP) [24]. SARNA and RdRP can be synthesized as two different amplicons or formulated as one *cis*-amplicon sequence in the lipid nanoparticle cargo. The ability to undergo several rounds of replication *in vivo* makes the SARNA vaccine more cost-effective than mRNA. However, SARNAs constructs are larger than those of mRNAs, and that feature may adversely alter the effectiveness of delivery. This concern is currently being addressed in phase 1, open-labeled trial NCT05155982. The study design includes 8 arms in which participants are administered 25 to 50 micrograms of SARNA-based COVAC-1 vaccine or placebo [25]. Two other SARNA vaccine candidates entered phase 2 clinical trials in the United Kingdom (randomized-controlled ISRCTN17072692, and NCT04758962) to assess the safety and measure the titers of vaccine-induced serum (IgG type) binding antibody responses to the SARS-CoV-2 S glycoprotein [26, 27].

Interestingly, both types of vaccines (mRNA and SARNA) elicited not only antigen-specific antibody responses but also antigen-specific T-cell responses, while SARNA elicited a stronger response at lower doses in mice [28]. A novel self-amplifying messenger ribonucleic acid (SAmRNA) trial by Gritstone Bio, Inc. is recruiting HIV-infected individuals to assess vaccine safety. Vaccines use a codon-optimized cassette covering multiple epitopes from the SARS-CoV-2 spike and non-spike proteins and additional T cell epitopes (NCT05435027) [29].

In lieu of fast changes in SARS-CoV-2 lineages, a variety of RNA vaccine reformulations may be needed to maintain emergency preparedness for future responses. A new development has recently been announced: the FDA granted emergency use authorizations (EUAs) to new formulations of both Pfizer-BioNTech and the Moderna COVID-19 vaccines. Authorized bivalent formulas, so-called "updated boosters" now contain two mRNA components of SARS-CoV-2 virus: the first is the originally approved (against lineage A of SARS-CoV-2); the second is common between the BA.4 and BA.5 lineages of the Omicron variant of SARS-CoV-2 [30]. Ongoing genomic surveillance of SARS-CoV-2 variants of concern allows real-time detection of immune escape mutations and prediction of vaccine breakthroughs [16].

3. Vaccines against human immunodeficiency virus infection

Human Immunodeficiency Virus (HIV) continues to present a serious global health threat since it made its appearance as a human-to-human transmitted pathogen, causing acquired immunodeficiency syndrome (AIDS) [31]. HIV1 and HIV2 are single-stranded positive-sense RNA retroviruses that are subdivided into several distinct classes [16]. HIV vaccine designs appeared to be the most challenging among other RNA viruses, due to frequent mutations, integration into the human genome, and a long latency phase [16].

There were more than two dozen HIV clinical trials conducted since early the 1990s that tested plasmid DNA-based protein vaccines as prophylactic or therapeutic types. These clinical trials were successful in phases 1 and 2; however, they were stopped in mid-phase 3 for futility by Data Safety Monitoring Board (DSMB) [32]. DSMB data analysis study did not find a statistically significant decrease in the number of HIV infections in the vaccine compared to placebo groups [33]. It was determined that the elicitation of humoral immune response was not robust enough to prevent infection or stop the progression of AIDS [34].

Numerous recombinant DNA-based vaccines were tested against several immunogenic epitopes (e.g., HIV protease, gag, env, gp120/140, or reverse transcriptase proteins) [35–37]. Various routes of administration (mucosal, intradermal, intravenous, and intramuscular) were also tested [33], and intramuscular injections were found to be the most efficacious. Recombinant DNA-based HIV vaccines generated only modest HIV-specific T cell and humoral responses, and that was insufficient for protection [38, 39]. Research studies on therapeutic vaccines continue to be performed. The randomized, double-blind, placebo-controlled dose escalation trimer-4571 vaccine (against HIV envelope protein) in combination with alum adjuvant has been the most widely reviewed study [40].

Ongoing challenges in HIV vaccine development include frequent HIV virus mutations that can lead to a glycan shield that covers HIV immunogens prompting Scripps Research Institute and Moderna's team to design a trimeric mRNA vaccine against HIV/AIDS (NCT05217641). The study focuses on recruiting participants who will be immunized with various doses of a modified trimeric vaccine composed of mRNA against glycan shields, CD4KO, and gp151 [41, 42]. Another phase 1 trial (NCT05001373) evaluates the safety and immunogenicity of two mRNA vaccine types after intraperitoneal administration. That trial aims to detect antigen-specific epitopes on CD4+ T cells and B cells in peripheral blood and in the germinal centers of secondary lymphoid organs [43]. Both mRNA trials are designed to induce Broadly Neutralizing Antibodies (BNAbs) in HIV-uninfected adult participants [44].

Different studies' interpretations differ in opinion with respect to the benefits and ability of HIV vaccines in activating endogenous single/double-stranded RNA sensing molecular machinery [45, 46]. It has been shown that in patients with advanced HIV infection, the immune system functions in absence of a sufficient amount of cytokine interferon-gamma (IFNG), and the innate immune branch often exhibits exaggerated responses to antigenic stimulation [47, 48]. Clinically, such responses are seen in the form of immune reconstitution inflammatory syndrome (IRIS) toward persistent antigens from previously treated opportunistic infections [49, 50]. Because they are not specific, vaccines can cause exaggerated systemic innate immune responses that lead to adverse events in immunocompromised individuals through activation and overexpression of TLR 3,7,8 OAS1–11, MDA1–5, IRFs, IFI, type 1 interferon genes, and the components of the inflammasome [49–52]. Adequate levels of interferon-gamma are necessary to establish appropriate virus-specific cytotoxic lymphocyte responses after therapeutic vaccination [53, 54]. IFNG is primarily produced by mature CD4+ T helper cells, which demonstrates low counts in immunocompromised individuals [55]. Therefore, the response to vaccines that are supplemented with adjuvants can be unpredictable [55]. The NCT04177355 trial evaluates the safety and immunogenicity of the HIV1BG505SOSIP.664gp140 vaccine in healthy HIV-uninfected adults [56]. This vaccine is formulated in combination with TLR-7/8 agonists and alum adjuvant (inflammasome activator). Yet, the safety of the vaccine/agonist/adjuvant combinations is needed to be assessed in HIV-infected populations to demonstrate clinical utility.

The major disadvantage of *in vitro*-transcribed mRNA vaccines is the unstable nature of mRNA molecules which often leads to their degradation by intracellular enzymes ribonucleases (i.e., RNases) [57]. mRNA synthesized by *in vitro* preparations can generate a small percentage of double-stranded RNAs that trigger activation of pathogen-associated molecular pathways through induction of interferon response genes [11]. The end result is enhanced mRNA degradation and a decrease in antigen production [58]. This is the main reason why formulations that used naked mRNA were unsuccessful [55]. Additionally, the poor thermal stability of mRNA vaccines requires product refrigeration. Those logistical constraints can present with problems during the distribution of the product in resource-limited settings (**Table 1**).

Perhaps the vaccine formulation for prophylactic and therapeutic vaccination should be different as the goal of the latter is to prevent the infection via various routes, and the former is to control localized viral replication. Researchers remain hopeful that novel self-amplifying vaccine formulations will lead to effective mosaic anti-HIV vaccines that completely interrupt HIV transmission and prevent subsequent infection [11].

4. Influenza vaccines

Influenza viruses are negative-sense, enveloped, segmented single-stranded RNA viruses that are encapsidated by nucleoproteins [59]. Several approved influenza vaccines were developed through recombinant DNA technology. These vaccines are reformulated annually based on predicted hemagglutinin (HA) and neuraminidase (NA) gene mutations (drifts and shifts). Constructs are delivered with baculovirus vector into host cells and recombinant HA protein is manufactured as a vaccine [60]. Influenza type A HA is subdivided into heterosubtypic groups 1–18, and influenza B - into 9. Several vaccines from four main biopharmaceutical companies are cleared by FDA: Fluad Quadrivalent and Flucelvax Quadrivalent are inactivated vaccines (Seqirus), Fluarix Quadrivalent is also inactivated vaccine (GlaxoSmithKline

Biologicals), and Flublok Quadrivalent is a recombinant influenza vaccine (Protein Sciences Corporation).

Many more vaccines are in clinical trials measuring primary outcomes as the humoral immune protection against surface viral proteins of seasonal avian influenza strains/subtypes/groups [61].

Pre-clinical trials in 2009 tested DNA plasmid carriers that contained genes that express viral antigens [62]. The poor success of those DNA-based vaccines may have been due to inefficient delivery of nucleic acids to cell nuclei and subsequent failure of DNA amplification in those target cells. Replication-competent and non-replicating adenoviral vectors offered improved delivery platform for influenza vaccines and achievement of systemic and mucosal immunity [63, 64]. As for mRNA and self-replicating RNA vaccines, they are delivered into the cytoplasm of cells but do not require nuclear translocation [65]. When formulated into lipid nanoparticles, RNA vaccines are efficiently delivered into the cytoplasm.

The first human clinical influenza mRNA-based trial employed a non-chemically modified mRNA construct, where the intent was to induce antibody titers against multivalent targets of four different influenza strains [66]. ModernaTX, Inc. is in recruitment of participants to evaluate modified mRNA-1647 to assess sero-responses in comparison to adjuvanted inactivated, quadrivalent seasonal influenza vaccine [67]. Subsequent vaccine goals include the development of multiplexed vaccine candidates into one dose of SARS-CoV-2, respiratory syncytial virus, or other formulations. Pfizer led a clinical research study of six SARNAs preparations of hemagglutinin antigens that were designed against four influenza strains. The proportion of participants achieving hemagglutination inhibition titers for each strain had been measured in the context of secondary outcomes [68]. It remains to be established if RNA vaccines will provide long-term protection with an established frequency of booster administration.

The global initiative on sharing all influenza data (GISAID) established the first repository of shared influenza sequences in 2006. GISAID has been instrumental for WHO and National Influenza Centers in providing bi-annual recommendations on strain selection for influenza vaccines [69]. Moreover, GISAID provides bioinformatics workspaces like FluSurver to allow scientists to perform assessments of the positions of novel mutations, changes in antigenic properties or glycosylation, and even predict viral susceptibility to drugs [70]. The geographical assessment of currently circulating strains can be visualized, as well as the phylogeny of current clades and the molecular clock of viral evolution (**Figure 1a, b**) [70]. For present strains of epidemiological importance, the frequency projections of currently circulating A/H3N2 clades are calculated from a fitness model based on the current frequency and estimated fitness [71]. The strain fitness is estimated by a combination of antigenic novelty and mutational load. Antigenic novelty is based on inferred measurements of antigenic advance from hemagglutination inhibition assay [71]. Mutational load is calculated by the number of amino acid mutations each strain carries at putative non-epitope sites relative to its most recent ancestor from the previous season (see **Figure 1** and pull down menus under Black “X” in: https://www.gisaid.org/epiflu-applications/influenza-genomic-epidemiology/).

a. Real-time tracking of influenza A/H1N1 evolution.

Top left: Rectangular phylogenetic tree of influenza A/H1N1 shows color-coded clades (by genotype). The black line represents linear regression of divergence. Black **X** represents an interactive drop-down menu with information about the date, specific nucleotides changes, amino acid changes, calculated divergence score, and potential vaccine selection. **Top right**: geographical distribution of A/H1N1 clades.

Bottom: Molecular clock representation of clades divergence since 2013, with an estimated rate of $3.7x10^{-3}$ substitutions per site per year.

b. Real-time tracking of influenza A/H3N2 evolution.

Top left: Rectangular phylogenetic tree of influenza A/H3N2 shows color-coded clades (by genotype). The black line represents linear regression of divergence. Black **X** represents interactive drop-down menu with information about the date, specific nucleotides changes, amino acid changes, calculated divergence score, and potential vaccine selection. **Top right**: geographical distribution of A/H3N2 clades.

Bottom: Molecular clock representation of clades divergence since 2013, with an estimated rate of $4.06x10^{-3}$ substitutions per site per year.

As more and more public health laboratories upload the sequencing results to GISAID, the global real-time tracking of influenza became possible. As a result, RNA vaccines can be re-designed just in a few days, and produced in just a few weeks.

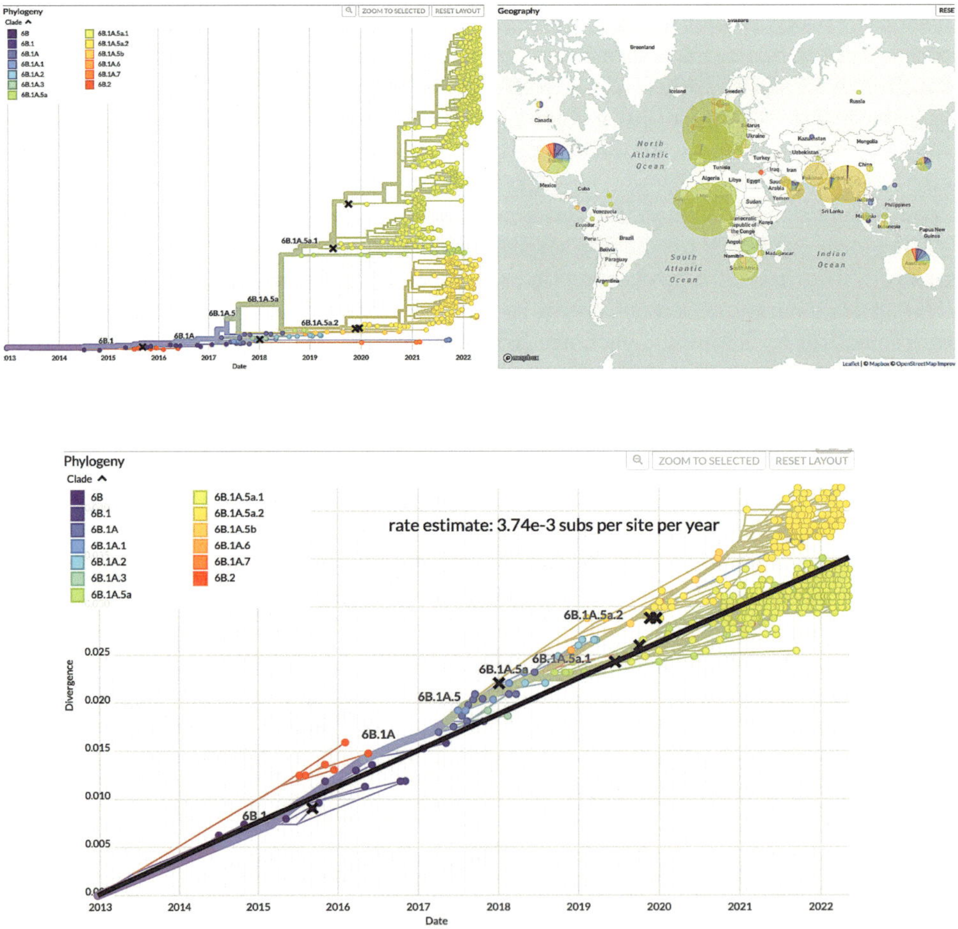

(a)

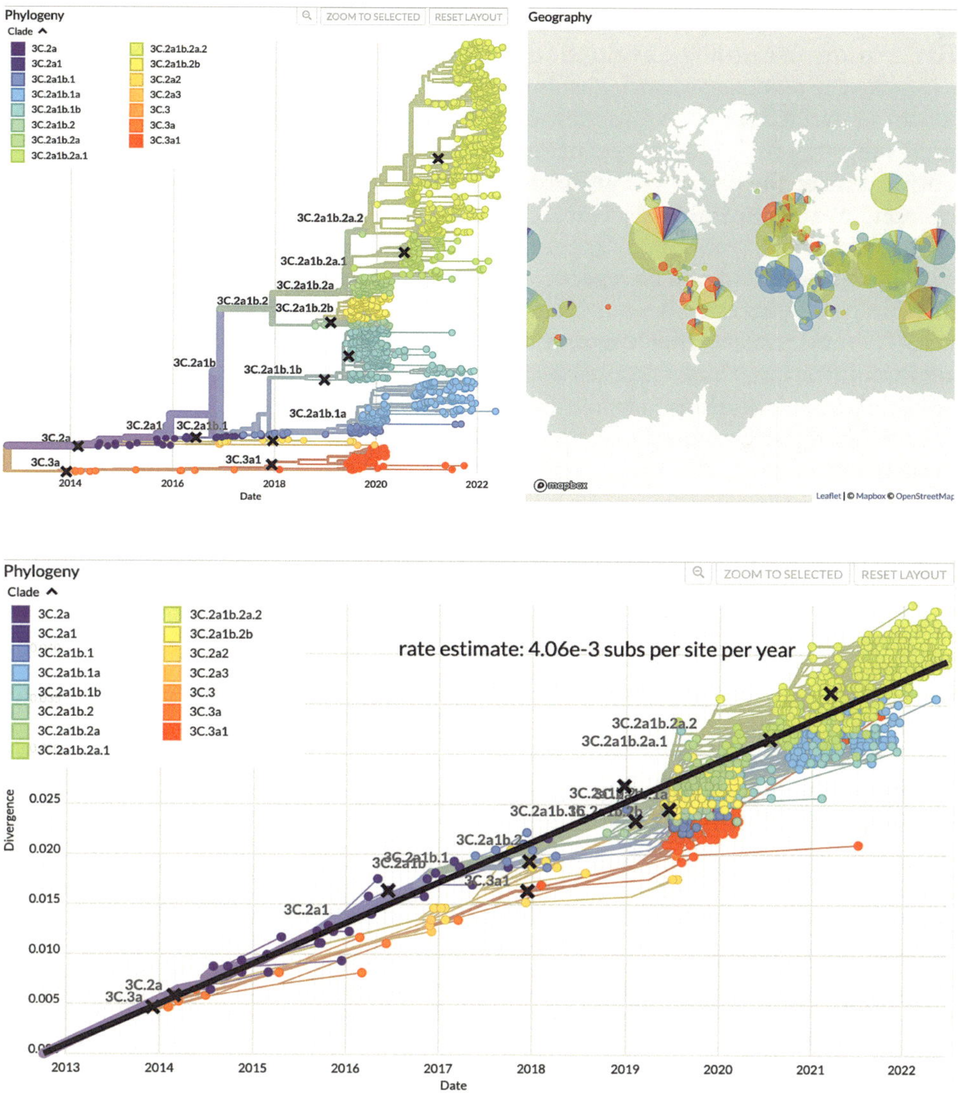

(b)

Figure 1.
Visualization of influenza phylogeny, geographical distribution, and divergence of clades.

5. Respiratory syncytial virus vaccines

The human respiratory syncytial virus (RSV) is a negative-strand RNA, enveloped, non-segmented virus of the order Mononegavirales, genus Pneumovirus and family Paramyxoviridae [72]. The human respiratory syncytial virus represents a significant public health burden in two main populations that includes young children and older adults. Previously, only passive immuno-prophylaxis with neutralizing antibodies was considered minimally protective against severe disease. The RSV-live attenuated vaccines did not prevent subsequent RSV disease [73]. Moreover, whole-virus inactivated vaccines were associated with enhanced respiratory disease in the lungs, presenting with monocytic eosinophilic pulmonary inflammation on histologic evaluation [74].

Despite the diversity of antigens, human RSV infection produces some serotypes that can be divided into two antigenic subgroups, with the RSV A being more diverse than B subgroup [75]. Elucidation of the atomic structure in conjunction with the identification of the fusion (F) glycoprotein was of critical importance for vaccine development and clinical trials. Unfortunately, these protein vaccines did not meet clinical expectations in robustness for preventing subsequent disease progression [76]. The development of a new generation of RSV-F protein, stabilized in the perfusion conformation, allowed GlaxoSmithKline and Medimmune to launch four phase-3 clinical trials testing pregnant mothers and infants [77]. Within 6 months after immunization, these vaccines were found to be protective against severe lower respiratory tract infections in infants and mothers [77].

An RSV-targeting recombinant virus-like particle vaccine trial (NCT04519073) conducted in Belgium demonstrated promising preliminary results of increased titers of micro-neutralizing antibodies against RSV A and B [78]. Additionally, a Phase 3 randomized, observer-blinded study evaluated the safety, tolerability, and immunogenicity of the mRNA-1345 (RSVictory) vaccine targeting RSV (NCT05127434) [79]. The vaccine was successfully tested in adults ≥50 years of age when administered alone or when co-administered with inactivated quadrivalent influenza vaccine (Afluria®) [80]). Outcome data will evaluate the percent of participants with sero-responses, who are defined by a ≥ 4-fold increase in RSV-A neutralizing antibody titer between one and six months after vaccination. This study has been conducted by ModernaTM, and the main outcome goal is to achieve long-term immunity to both infections. These vaccines are yet to show reliable prophylactic and therapeutic efficacy.

6. Combination vaccines against parainfluenza type 3 virus (PIV3) and human Metapneumovirus (HMPV)

Like RSV, PIV is also a negative-strand RNA virus from the Paramyxoviridae family and Paramyxovirinae subfamily. Bi-directional high-throughput RNA sequencing technology elucidated several types of parainfluenzas (1–5), with PIV3 as most predominant [81]. Another, more recently identified member of the order Mononegavirales, family Paramyxoviridae, subfamily Pneumovirinae is a human metapneumovirus (HMPV) [82]. HMPV became a part of infectious disease genomic surveillance after development of whole-genome tiled amplicon sequencing technology. This methodology allowed the identification of two major phylogenetic subtypes of HMPV, each containing two sublineages (A1, A2, B1, B2) [83, 84]. The use of this new knowledge in vaccine manufacturing led to multi-viral vaccine research and development.

Human subfamilies (Paramyxovirinae and Pneumovirinae) are known to cause hospital-acquired infections, infections in young and elderly adults, and pneumonia in immunocompromised individuals [85]. Antiviral medication or vaccinations against these globally spread viral infections, including multiple re-infections that occur throughout life, did not exist until recently. Two clinical trials conducted by Moderna TX are recruiting participants to assess the safety, reactogenicity, and Immunogenicity of the mRNA-1653 vaccine. This is a combined design against PIV and HMPV, which will be tested in healthy adults (NCT03392389) and children 12 to 59 months of age (NCT04144348) [86, 87]. If these trials are successful, other Paramyxoviridae infections can be targeted with the same polyvalent vaccine design.

7. Chikungunya and dengue viruses' vaccine trials

Chikungunya, Dengue, and Zika viruses are transmitted by mosquitos of the *Aedes* genus. These infections had little attention in Western World prior to travel-related epidemics spreading from tropical countries of equatorial Africa, South America, India, or the Polynesian region.

The mosquito-borne Chikungunya fever is caused by RNA arbovirus that belongs to the alphavirus genus of the family Togaviridae. Patients usually present with relatively mild disease; however, debilitating chronic arthritis has been reported in some patients who recover from the infection [88].

Phase 1 and 2 clinical trials of Chikungunya virus-like recombinant protein vaccines (aluminum hydroxide-adjuvanted) have been completed [89–91]. One study, conducted by Emergent BioSolutions (PXVX0317) reported promising results related to satisfactory safety outcomes and sufficient neutralizing antibody titer responses (NCT0348369; NCT03992872) [92]. Phase 3 was initiated in August 2022, and the focus was to test PXVX031 in adults ≥65 years of age [93].

DNA-based vaccines have been designed and tested (based on mumps and rubella viral vectors), but those vaccines failed to demonstrate long-term immunogenicity [94]. Two years before the COVID-19 pandemic, Moderna launched the first Phase 1 trial of the mRNA-1388 vaccine and subsequently the second trial of mRNA-1944 [95, 96]. Although these trials were interrupted by the COVID-19 pandemic, preliminary results showed favorable tolerability of mRNAs in healthy volunteers. mRNA-1388 is a prophylactic vaccine that consists of a single mRNA encoding the full native structural polyprotein (C-E3-E2-6k-E1 peptides). This polyprotein is naturally processed into C and E structural viral proteins that assemble into viral-like particles before being released from cells [97]. mRNA-1944 encodes the heavy and light chains of the Chikungunya antibody formulated in proprietary lipid nanoparticles and can be used as biotherapeutics [97]. More information about these vaccines and trial designs can be found in the archives of the United States Security and Exchange Commission reports [97].

Sequencing of the full 10 kB Chikungunya virus genome is important for epidemiological investigation and genomic surveillance; however, few Public Health Laboratories are pursuing these investigations [98]. Understanding genetic diversity and rates of *de novo* mutations will allow estimates of higher and lower fitness of circulating variants (those that have sufficient fitness to cause epidemics and those that can be naturally purified during transmission bottlenecks) [98, 99]. Similar analogies can be made with the 10.7-kB ribonucleic acid virus Dengue. The incidence of Dengue disease is increasing globally and is attributed to the exportation of the disease from tropical countries via tourism and inefficient mosquito controls. Significant concerns about the spread of this emerging disease, as well as potential solutions are elucidated in comprehensive reviews on dengue vaccine development [100–103]. The development of effective vaccines and mandatory vaccination of international travelers has already proven to be the most effective way in preventing the transmission of vector-borne diseases like yellow fever [104]. Thus, vaccination certificates may be required in the future for travelers as a condition of entry to specific countries, and this would facilitate safer international travel.

8. Zika virus vaccines

Zika is an eleven-kilobases-long single-stranded positive-sense RNA virus. Zika's genome encodes for one open-reading frame, which is translated into 20 functional proteins. There are seven nonstructural and 13 structural proteins, including pre-membrane, envelope, and capsid. Like most flaviviruses, Zika is transmitted by mosquitos. Intercontinental travel has facilitated Zika virus spread out of Africa, as well as it is being spread from human to human via sexual contact. Pregnancy, in conjunction with gestational Zika infection, is strongly associated with microcephaly and other congenital abnormalities in newborns. Preventing congenital Zika infections has been the subject of vaccine research in animal models [105].

Pre-clinical Zika studies with the modified-nucleoside mRNA vaccines have been designed to target the envelope and pre-membrane proteins [106]. Recently initiated Moderna's phase 1 and 2 human clinical trials have shown a near 90% seroconversion rate in adult participants after booster vaccination [107]. Phase 2 of this study is expected to be completed in 2024, with the primary outcome measure focusing on systemic reactogenicity while reducing adverse events, and achieving measurable serum-neutralizing antibodies against Zika virus [108].

Various formulations of SARNA vaccine studies in animal models have been compared with the efficacy of DNA and mRNA vaccines [109]. SARNAs have shown to be more effective in smaller doses compared to the other vaccines. One reason is attributed to the double-stranded SARNA being able to induce innate immune interferon type 1/2 responses, which serve as an endogenous adjuvant. This has been proposed to eliminate the administration of a second dose that is required for mRNA vaccines. In comparison, the second and third exposures to DNA vaccines elicit host immune response against the vectors that contain the vaccines' DNA (**Table 1**). Conversely, this is not known side-effect for mRNA or SARNAs because the majority of those vaccines are encapsulated into non-immunogenic neutral or charged lipid nanoparticles [110]. Seventy other DNA, RNA, and conventional Zika-vaccine studies are currently registered with clinicaltrials.org in the assessment of safety and preliminary efficacy (phases 1 and 2). Future studies are required to demonstrate which vaccine could be more robust, providing longer-lasting immunity against Zika infection.

9. Rabies virus vaccines

The rabies virus is an RNA virus transmitted through mammalian vectors. The genome of the rabies virus encodes 5 proteins (N, P, M, G, and L), and the sequencing of the single-stranded RNA genome classified the viral structure within the Lyssavirus family. Due to the neurotropic properties of the virus and a lack of effective treatment, rabies exposure, if not immediately addressed, is lethal in humans and other mammals within three weeks from infection [111]. Furthermore, vaccine portfolios have not significantly advanced, and that may be in part due to the endemic and sporadic nature of the disease. While DNA vaccines against rabies have been developed, they have proven to be poorly immunogenic in humans [112]. Thus, conventional types of inactivated rabies virus vaccines (RabAvert, Rabipur, Imovax, etc.) are most common for vaccination of individuals in specific professions who are at high risk of rabies exposure [111].

mRNA rabies vaccines CureVac and CV7201 entered phase 1 clinical trial in order to assess their safety and reactogenicity [113, 114]. These mRNA vaccines also encode rabies virus glycoprotein G and have shown promise to be safe and effective as a pre- and early post-exposure prophylactic vaccine for humans (NCT03713086; NCT02241135). Several novel self-amplifying RNA (SARNA) have been tested in combination with diverse nanoparticle formulations. Preclinical studies of proprietary cationic nanoemulsion-formulated glycoprotein G-encoding self-amplifying RNA (RG-SAM [CNE]) showed that the vaccine was well tolerated following multiple intramuscular injections in animals [112]. The rabies SARNA is a virus glycoprotein G RNA that showed promising results in phase 1 clinical studies through protecting neutralizing antibody responses (IgM and IgG) against viral glycoprotein. SARNA vaccines are well tolerated and cause mild side effects comparable to those in conventional vaccines trial (GlaxoSmithKline, NCT04062669) [115]. Establishing clinical efficacy is the next step for this type of SARNA vaccines, as they hold great promise to become valuable pre-exposure prophylactics. SARNA technology offers distinct advantages because they are highly amenable to mass- *in vitro*- transcription in GMP-level facilities.

10. Ebola virus disease vaccines

Ebola is a single-stranded, negative-sense RNA virus that causes the Ebola virus disease. Ebola is subdivided into five immunologically different subspecies based on surface envelope glycoprotein spikes and the virion proteins of nucleocapsid [116]. UCSC Genome Browser and GISAID contain the most comprehensive genomic information on Ebola subspecies sequence variations and phylogeography [117, 118].

More than four dozen vaccine trials were initiated after the Ebola outbreak of 2014 [119]. At least half of them were DNA-based transgenes, delivered with non-replicative viral vectors like Venezuelan equine encephalitis virus, human replication-defective adenovirus, recombinant chimpanzee adenovirus type 3, modified vaccinia strain Ankara, or Kunjin replicon virus-like particle vaccine. The other vaccine trials utilized replicative vectors, including human parainfluenza virus type 3-based vaccine, recombinant vesicular stomatitis virus-based vaccine (rVSV-EBOV), recombinant rabies virus, or recombinant cytomegalovirus. All of these vaccines were designed against envelope spike glycoproteins [120].

The first Ebola vaccine (rVSV-ZEBOV, Merk) was approved in the United States in 2019 and had been used in the 2018 Ebola epidemic in the Democratic Republic of the Congo as part of clinical trials. Subsequently, it had been used under criteria for compassionate use that included children and pregnant women [121]. rVSV-ZEBOV showed the ability to generate protective immunity in a form of anti-glycoprotein immunoglobulin G antibody titers that lasted at least 2 years of observation [122]. Several other DNA-based vaccines are being tested by Inovio Pharmaceuticals via routes of prime intramuscular injection with subsequent boost electroporation [123]. Electroporation is less invasive; however, it requires a specialized medical device to deliver brief electrical pulses during intradermal gene transfer [124]. Challenges remain with DNA vaccine platforms. These challenges include immune response to viral vectors after booster vaccination, safety concerns about replication-capable viral cargo (e.g., human genome integration), and slow optimization of antigen sequences to make multivalent vaccines against all sub-strains of the Ebola virus (**Table 1**).

mRNA vaccines can respond to these challenges quicker because the manufacturing process and formulations allow multi-sequence delivery and, therefore, avoids safety issues associated with booster immunization. The lipid nanoparticle (LNP) encapsulation technology and the design of glycoprotein mRNA with post-transcriptional modifications have the potential to exhibit durable immune responses in pre-clinical and phase 1 studies [125]. Due to lower doses requirement, and lower cost, SARNA vaccines may have a higher potential to rapidly respond to future Ebola outbreaks. Like DNA vaccines, SARNAs are stable and can be delivered intradermally via electroporation. Non-human primate experiments showed that SARNA induces sufficient protective responses against Ebola after a single primed immunization [126]. Future expectations are that SARNA vaccines will be successfully delivered with electroporation (intradermal) and will not require boost immunization.

11. Future directions

Epidemics caused by genetically recombined or mutated RNA viruses will continue to evolve and pose health threats locally and globally. Because of this, RNA vaccinology will continue to strive to develop new manufacturing processes to improve RNA transcript stability by incorporating modified synthetic nucleotides during *in vitro* transcription, optimizing delivery formulations, and adjusting the adjuvants' potency. Additionally, next-generation viral genotyping conducted by CDC and Public Health Laboratories will provide real-time pathogen surveillance data for rapid modifications and manufacturing of RNA vaccines. Mosaic vaccines against multiple viral strains or multi-pathogen vaccines are a goal that needs to be achieved to prevent pandemics, epidemics, and endemic infections.

Acknowledgements

IVS is sponsored by APHL/CDC COVID-19 Laboratory Associate Fellowship grant, and Ronald H. Laessig Memorial Newborn Screening Fellowship fund.

Conflict of interest

None declared.

Abbreviations

GISAID	global initiative on sharing all influenza data
TLR	Toll-Like Receptor
IRF	Interferon regulatory factor
IFI	Interferon alpha inducible protein
OAS	2′-5′-Oligoadenylate synthetases
GMP	Good manufacturing practice
MDA5	melanoma differentiation-associated protein 5
UCSC	University of California Santa Cruz

Author details

Irina Vlasova-St. Louis[1,2]* and Jude Abadie[3,4]

1 Individualized Genomics and Health Program, Johns Hopkins University, Baltimore, MD, USA

2 Molecular Branch of Newborn Screening Program, Texas Department of State Health Services, Austin, Texas, USA

3 El Paso Public Health Laboratory, USA

4 Texas Tech University Health Sciences Center El Paso, USA

*Address all correspondence to: stlouis.irina@gmail.com

References

[1] HHS.gov. Vaccine Types. 2021. Available from: https://www.hhs.gov/immunization/basics/types/index.html [Accessed: 17 July 2022]

[2] McFarland EJ, Karron RA, Muresan P, et al. Live-attenuated respiratory syncytial virus vaccine with M2-2 deletion and with small hydrophobic noncoding region is highly immunogenic in children. The Journal of Infectious Diseases. 2020;**221**:2050-2059

[3] Rodrigues AF, Soares HR, Guerreiro MR, et al. Viral vaccines and their manufacturing cell substrates: New trends and designs in modern vaccinology. Biotechnology Journal. 2015;**10**:1329-1344

[4] D'Amico C, Fontana F, Cheng R, et al. Development of vaccine formulations: Past, present, and future. Drug Deliv. Translational Research. 2021;**11**:765-777

[5] Leitner WW, Ying H, Restifo NP. DNA and RNA-based vaccines: Principles, progress and prospects. Vaccine. 1999;**18**:765-777

[6] Plotkin S, Robinson JM, Cunningham G, et al. The complexity and cost of vaccine manufacturing – An overview. Vaccine. 2017;**35**:4064-4071

[7] Rosa SS, Prazeres DMF, Azevedo AM, et al. mRNA vaccines manufacturing: Challenges and bottlenecks. Vaccine. 2021;**39**:2190-2200

[8] Suzuki Y, Ishihara H. Difference in the lipid nanoparticle technology employed in three approved siRNA (Patisiran) and mRNA (COVID-19 vaccine) drugs. Drug Metabolism and Pharmacokinetics. 2021;**41**:1-7

[9] Maruggi G, Ulmer JB, Rappuoli R, et al. Self-amplifying mRNA-Based Vaccine Technology and Its Mode of Action. Berlin: Springer Berlin Heidelberg, 2021. Epub ahead of print 2021. DOI: 10.1007/82_2021_233

[10] Bloom K, van den Berg F, Arbuthnot P. Self-amplifying RNA vaccines for infectious diseases. Gene Therapy. 2021;**28**:117-129

[11] Mu Z, Haynes BF, Cain DW. HIV mRNA vaccines—Progress and future paths. Vaccine. 2021;**9**:1-22

[12] Dolgin E. The tangled history of mRNA vaccines. Nature. 2021;**597**:318-324

[13] Tenchov R, Bird R, Curtze AE, et al. Lipid nanoparticles from liposomes to mRNA vaccine delivery, a landscape of research diversity and advancement. ACS Nano. 2021;**15**:16982-17015

[14] Zhou Y, Jiang S, Du L. Prospects for a MERS-CoV spike vaccine. Expert Review of Vaccines. 2018;**17**:677-686

[15] Unchwaniwala N, Ahlquist P. Coronavirus dons a new crown. Science. 2020;**369**:1306-1307

[16] Vlasova-St. Louis I, Gorzalski A, Pandori M. Diagnostic Applications for RNA- Seq Technology and Transcriptome Analyses in Human Diseases Caused by RNA Viruses. In: Applications of RNA-Seq in Biology and Medicine. IntechOpen; pp. 122-138

[17] Kaur SP, Gupta V. COVID-19 vaccine: A comprehensive status report. Virus Research. 2020;**288**:1-12

[18] ModernaTX Inc. Dose-Confirmation Study to Evaluate the Safety, Reactogenicity, and

Immunogenicity of mRNA-1273 COVID-19 Vaccine in Adults Aged 18 Years and Older. NCT04405076. Epub ahead of print 2020. Available from: https://clinicaltrials.gov/ct2/show/NCT04405076

[19] Pfizer, BioNTech SE. A Study to Evaluate Safety, Tolerability, & Immunogenicity of Multiple Formulations of BNT162b2 Against COVID-19 in Healthy Adults. 2021. Available from: https://clinicaltrials.gov/ct2/show/NCT04816669?term=BNT162b2&draw=2&rank=3

[20] Wang M, Wen W, Zhou M, et al. Meta-analysis of risk of myocarditis after messenger RNA COVID-19 vaccine. The American Journal of Cardiology. 2022;**167**:155-157

[21] Bottazzi ME, Strych U, Hotez PJ, et al. Coronavirus vaccine-associated lung immunopathology-what is the significance? Microbes and Infection. 2020;**22**:403-404

[22] Siolos A, Gartzonika K, Tigas S. Thyroiditis following vaccination against COVID-19: Report of two cases and review of the literature. Metabolism Open. 2021;**12**:1-2

[23] Maruggi G, Mallett CP, Westerbeck JW, et al. A self-amplifying mRNA SARS-CoV-2 vaccine candidate induces safe and robust protective immunity in preclinical models. Molecular Therapy. 2022;**30**:1897-1912

[24] de Alwis R, Gan ES, Chen S, et al. A single dose of self-transcribing and replicating RNA-based SARS-CoV-2 vaccine produces protective adaptive immunity in mice. Molecular Therapy. 2021;**29**:1970-1983

[25] ClinicalTrials.gov. A Clinical Trial of COVAC-1 in Generally Healthy Adults. NCT05155982. Epub ahead of print 2021. Available from: https://clinicaltrials.gov/ct2/show/NCT05155982

[26] Medical Research Council Clinical Trials Unit at UCL (UK). Clinical trial to Assess the Safety of a Coronavirus Vaccine in Healthy Men and Women. ISRCTN17072692. Epub ahead of print 2020. Available from: https://www.isrctn.com/ISRCTN17072692

[27] GlaxoSmithKline. A Study of the Safety of and Immune Response to Varying Doses of a Vaccine Against COVID-19 in Healthy Adults. NCT04758962. 2021. Available from: https://clinicaltrials.gov/ct2/show/NCT04758962

[28] Rappaport AR, Hong S-J, Scallan CD, et al. Low-dose self-amplifying mRNA COVID-19 vaccine drives strong protective immunity in non-human primates against SARS-CoV-2 infection. Nature Communications. 2022;**13**:3289

[29] ClinicalTrials.gov. Study of Self-Amplifying Messenger Ribonucleic Acid (samRNA) Vaccines Against COVID-19 in Healthy Adults and People Living With Human Immunodeficiency Virus (HIV). NCT05435027. Epub ahead of print 2022. Available from: https://clinicaltrials.gov/ct2/show/NCT05435027

[30] FDA. Coronavirus (COVID-19) Update: FDA Authorizes Moderna, Pfizer- BioNTech Bivalent COVID-19 Vaccines for Use as a Booster Dose. Epub ahead of print 2022. Available from: https://www.fda.gov/news-events/press- announcements/coronavirus-covid-19-update-fda-authorizes-moderna- pfizer-biontech-bivalent-covid-19-vaccines-use#:~:text=Today%2C%20the%20U.S.%20Food%20and,following%20primary%20or%20booster%20vaccination

[31] van Wyngaard A, Whiteside A. AIDS and COVID-19 in southern Africa. African Journal of AIDS Research. 2021;**20**:17-124

[32] D'haese S, Lacroix C, Garcia F, Plana M, Ruta S, Vanham G, et al. Off the beaten path: Novel mRNA-nanoformulations for therapeutic vaccination against HIV. Journal of Controlled Release. 2021;**330**:1016-1033

[33] Hokello J, Sharma AL, Tyagi M. An update on the HIV DNA vaccine strategy. Vaccine. 2021;**9**:605

[34] Flynn NM, Forthal DN, Harro CD, et al. Placebo-controlled phase 3 trial of a recombinant glycoprotein 120 vaccine to prevent HIV-1 infection. The Journal of Infectious Diseases. 2005;**191**:654-655

[35] Hemachandra A, Puls RL, Sirivichayakul S, et al. An HIV-1 clade a/E DNA prime, recombinant fowlpox virus boost vaccine is safe, but non-immunogenic in a randomized phase 1/11a trial in Thai volunteers at low risk of HIV infection. Human Vaccines. 2010;**6**:835-840

[36] Mehendale S, Van Lunzen J, Clumeck N, et al. A phase 1 study to evaluate the safety and immunogenicity of a recombinant HIV type 1 subtype C adeno-associated virus vaccine. AIDS Research and Human Retroviruses. 2008;**24**:873-880

[37] Sanders RW, Derking R, Cupo A, et al. A next-generation cleaved, soluble HIV-1 Env trimer, BG505 SOSIP.664 gp140, expresses multiple epitopes for broadly neutralizing but not non-neutralizing antibodies. PLoS Pathogens. 2013;**9**:e1003618

[38] Vardas E, Kaleebu P, Bekker LG, et al. A phase 2 study to evaluate the safety and immunogenicity of a recombinant hiv type 1 vaccine based on adeno-associated virus. AIDS Research and Human Retroviruses. 2010;**26**:933-942

[39] Pitisuttithum P, Nitayaphan S, Chariyalertsak S, et al. Late boosting of the RV144 regimen with AIDSVAX B/E and ALVAC-HIV in HIV-uninfected Thai volunteers: A double-blind, randomised controlled trial. Lancet HIV. 2020;**7**:e238–e248

[40] ClinicalTrials.gov. Evaluation of Trimer 4571 Therapeutic Vaccination in Adults Living With HIV on Suppressive Antiretroviral Therapy (NETI). NCT04985760. Epub ahead of print 2021. Available from: https://clinicaltrials.gov/ct2/show/NCT04985760

[41] Steichen JM, Kulp DW, Tokatlian T, et al. HIV vaccine design to target germline precursors of glycan-dependent broadly neutralizing antibodies. Immunity. 2016;**45**:483-496

[42] Wagh K, Hahn BH, Korber B. Hitting the sweet spot: Exploiting HIV-1 glycan shield for induction of broadly neutralizing antibodies. Current Opinion in HIV AIDS. 2020;**15**:267-274

[43] ClinicalTrials.gov. A Phase 1 Study to Evaluate the Safety and Immunogenicity of eOD-GT8 60mer mRNA Vaccine (mRNA-1644) and Core-g28v2 60mer mRNA Vaccine (mRNA-1644v2-Core). NCT05001373. Epub ahead of print 2021. Available from: https://clinicaltrials.gov/ct2/show/NCT05001373

[44] ClinicalTrials.gov. A Clinical Trial to Evaluate the Safety and Immunogenicity of BG505 MD39.3, BG505 MD39.3 gp151, and BG505 MD39.3 gp151 CD4KO HIV Trimer mRNA Vaccines in Healthy, HIV-uninfected Adult Participants. NCT05217641. Epub ahead of print 2022. Available from: https://clinicaltrials.gov/ct2/show/NCT05217641

[45] Seddiki N, French M. COVID-19 and HIV-associated immune reconstitution inflammatory syndrome: Emergence of pathogen-specific immune responses adding fuel to the fire. Frontiers in Immunology. 2021;**12**:1-8

[46] Coffman RL, Sher A, Seder RA. Vaccine adjuvants: Putting innate immunity to work. Immunity. 2010;**33**:492-503

[47] Mohei H, Kellampalli U, Vlasova-St. Louis I. Immune reconstitution disorders: Spotlight on interferons. International Journal of Biomedical Investigation. 2019;**2**:1-21

[48] Kellampalli U, Mohei H, Vlasova-St. Louis I. The role of cytokines and cellular receptors in the tuberculosis- associated immune reconstitution inflammatory syndrome. Journal of Infectious Diseases & Case Reports. 2021;**1**:1-5

[49] Vlasova-St Louis I, Musubire AK, Meya DB, et al. Transcriptomic biomarker pathways associated with death in HIV-infected patients with cryptococcal meningitis. BMC Medical Genomics. 2021;**14**:2-14

[50] Vlasova-St. Louis I, Chang CC, Shahid S, et al. Transcriptomic predictors of paradoxical cryptococcosis-associated immune reconstitution inflammatory syndrome. Open Forum Infectious Diseases. 2018;**5**:1-10

[51] Brienze VMS, André JC, Liso E, Vlasova-St. Louis I. Cryptococcal immune reconstitution inflammatory syndrome: From blood and cerebrospinal fluid biomarkers to treatment approaches. Life. 2021;**11**:2-18

[52] Kellampalli U, Mohei H, Vlasova-St. Louis I. Immune restoration disorders in patients with AIDS and tuberculosis: Novel treatment approaches. ACTA Science Microbiology. 2021;**4**:133-139

[53] Bejanyan N, Vlasova-St Louis I, Mohei H, et al. Cytomegalovirus-specific immunity recovers more slowly after cord blood transplantation compared with matched sibling donor allogeneic transplantation. Transplant Cell Therapy. 2021;**27**:187.e1-187.e4

[54] Kellampalli U, Mohei H, Vlasova-St. Louis I. Kinetics of immune reconstitution and immune complications after cell and organ transplantation. Integration Cancer Science Therapy. 2020;**7**:2-6

[55] ClinicalTrials.gov. iHIVARNA Clinical Trial in HIV Infected Individuals (iHIVARNA-01). NCT02888756. Epub ahead of print 2016. Available from: https://clinicaltrials.gov/ct2/show/NCT02888756

[56] ClinicalTrials.gov. Evaluating the Safety and Immunogenicity of HIV-1 BG505 SOSIP.664 gp140 With TLR Agonist and/or Alum Adjuvants in Healthy, HIV-uninfected Adults. NCT04177355. Epub ahead of print 2019. Available from: https://clinicaltrials.gov/ct2/show/NCT04177355

[57] Liu T, Liang Y, Huang L. Development and delivery systems of mRNA vaccines. Frontiers in Bioengineering and Biotechnology. 2021;**9**:1-10

[58] Pardi N, Kariko K, Hogan M, et al. Generating an anti-HIV vaccine using nucleoside-modified mRNA encoding envelope. AIDS Research and Human Retroviruses. 2014;**30**:25-41

[59] Bouvier NM, Palese P. The biology of influenza viruses. Vaccine. 2008;**26**:49-53

[60] Fabre LL, Arrías PN, Masson T, et al. Baculovirus-derived vectors for immunization and therapeutic applications. In: Emerging and Reemerging Viral Pathogens. Vol. 2. Applied Virology Approaches Related

to Human, Animal and Environmental Pathogens. Cambridge MA: Academic Press; 2019. pp. 198-224

[61] Nachbagauer R, Feser J, Naficy A, et al. A chimeric hemagglutinin-based universal influenza virus vaccine approach induces broad and long-lasting immunity in a randomized, placebo-controlled phase I trial. Nature Medicine. 2021;**27**:106-110

[62] ClinicalTrials.gov. DNA-based Influenza Vaccine in the Elderly. NCT01587131. Epub ahead of print 2012. Available from: https://www.clinicaltrials.gov/ct2/show/NCT01587131

[63] Matsuda K, Migueles SA, Huang J, et al. A replication-competent adenovirus-vectored influenza vaccine induces durable systemic and mucosal immunity. The Journal of Clinical Investigation. 2021;**131**:1-15

[64] Kerstetter LJ, Buckley S, Bliss CM, Coughlan L, Ben-Yedidia T. Adenoviral Vectors as Vaccines for Emerging Avian Influenza Viruses. 2021;**11**:1-27

[65] Rockman S, Laurie KL, Parkes S, et al. New technologies for influenza vaccines. Microorganisms. 2020;**8**:1-20

[66] ClinicalTrials.gov. A Study to Evaluate the Safety, Reactogenicity and Immunogenicity of Vaccine CVSQIV in Healthy Adults. Epub ahead of print 2022. Available from: https://clinicaltrials.gov/ct2/show/NCT05252338

[67] ClinicalTrials.gov. A Study of Modified mRNA Vaccines in Healthy Adults. NCT05397223. Epub ahead of print 2022. Available from: https://clinicaltrials.gov/ct2/show/NCT05397223

[68] ClinicalTrials.gov. A Study to Evaluate Self-Amplifying Ribonucleic Acid (RNA) Vaccine Preparations Against Influenza. NCT05227001. Epub ahead of print 2022. Available from: https://clinicaltrials.gov/ct2/show/NCT05227001

[69] Shu Y, McCauley J. GISAID: Global initiative on sharing all influenza data – From vision to reality. Eurosurveillance. 2017;**22**:30494

[70] GISAID. H3N2 Influenza A Genomic Epidemiology. 2006. Available from: https://www.gisaid.org/epiflu-applications/influenza-genomic-epidemiology/ [Accessed: 2 July 2022]

[71] Huddleston J, Barnes JR, Rowe T, et al. Integrating genotypes and phenotypes improves long-term forecasts of seasonal influenza a/H3N2 evolution. eLife. 2020;**9**:1-38

[72] Battles MB, McLellan JS. Respiratory syncytial virus entry and how to block it. Nature Reviews Microbiology. 2019;**17**:233-245

[73] Ruckwardt TJ, Morabito KM, Graham BS. Immunological lessons from respiratory syncytial virus vaccine development. Immunity. 2019;**51**:429-442

[74] Kim HW, Canchola JG, Brandt CD, et al. Respiratory syncytial virus disease in infants despite prior administration of antigenic inactivated vaccine. American Journal of Epidemiology. 1969;**89**:422-434

[75] Collins PL, Fearns R, Graham BS. Respiratory syncytial virus: Virology, reverse genetics, and pathogenesis of disease. Current Topics in Microbiology and Immunology. 2013;**372**:3-27

[76] Mejias A, Rodríguez-Fernández R, Oliva S, Peeples ME, Ramilo O. The journey to a respiratory syncytial virus vaccine. Annals of Allergy, Asthma and Immunology. 2020;**125**:36-46

[77] Ginsburg AS, Srikantiah P. Respiratory syncytial virus: Promising progress against a leading cause of pneumonia. The Lancet Global Health. 2021;**9**:e1644–e1645

[78] ClinicalTrials.gov. Phase 1 Study to Evaluate the Safety and Immunogenicity of a Candidate Vaccine Against Respiratory Syncytial Virus. NCT05001373

[79] ClinicalTrials.gov. A Study to Evaluate the Safety and Efficacy of mRNA-1345 Vaccine Targeting Respiratory Syncytial Virus (RSV) in Adults ≥60 Years of Age. NCT05127434. Epub ahead of print 2022. Available from: https://clinicaltrials.gov/ct2/show/NCT05127434

[80] ClinicalTrials.gov. A Study of mRNA-1345 Vaccine Targeting Respiratory Syncytial Virus (RSV) in Adults ≥50 Years of Age (RSVictory) [Internet]. NCT05330975. 2022. Available from: https://clinicaltrials.gov/ct2/show/NCT05330975

[81] Wignall-Fleming EB, Hughes DJ, Vattipally S, et al. Analysis of paramyxovirus transcription and replication by high-throughput sequencing. Journal of Virology. 2019;**93**:1-39

[82] Burrell CJ, Howard CR, Murphy FA. Fenner and White's Medical Virology. Fifth Edition. Cambridge MA: Academic Press; 2016

[83] Tulloch RL, Kok J, Carter I, et al. An amplicon-based approach for the whole-genome sequencing of human metapneumovirus. Viruses. 2021;**13**:1-11

[84] Kamau E, Oketch JW, De Laurent ZR, et al. Whole Genome Sequencing and Phylogenetic Analysis of Human Metapneumovirus Strains from Kenya and Zambia. BMC Genomics. 2020;**21**:1-10

[85] Kakiuchi S, Tsuji M, Nishimura H, et al. Human parainfluenza virus type 3 infections in patients with hematopoietic stem cell transplants: The mode of nosocomial infections and prognosis. Japanese Journal of Infectious Diseases. 2018;**71**:109-115

[86] ClinicalTrials.gov. Safety, Reactogenicity, and Immunogenicity of mRNA-1653 in Healthy Adults. NCT03392389. Epub ahead of print 2021. Available from: https://clinicaltrials.gov/ct2/show/NCT03392389

[87] ClinicalTrials.gov. Safety and Immunogenicity of mRNA-1653, a Combined Human Metapneumovirus (hMPV) and Parainfluenza Virus Type 3 (PIV3) Vaccine, in Healthy Adults, and Children 12 to 59 Months of Age With Serologic Evidence of Prior Exposure. Epub ahead of print 2022. Available from: https://www.clinicaltrials.gov/ct2/show/NCT04144348

[88] Bukhari SR, Mahmood SU, Jamal AM, et al. Chikungunya on the move- reflection from Pakistan. International Journal of Community Medicine and Public Health. 2018;**5**:1676– 1678

[89] ClinicalTrials.gov. Chikungunya Vaccine (V184) Study in Previously Exposed Adults (V184-006). NCT03807843. Epub ahead of print 2019. Available from: https://clinicaltrials.gov/ct2/show/results/NCT03807843

[90] ClinicalTrials.gov. Safety, Tolerability and Long-term Immunogenicity of Different Formulations of a Chikungunya Vaccine (V184-005). NCT03635086. 2018. Available from: https://clinicaltrials.gov/ct2/show/NCT03635086

[91] ClinicalTrials.gov. Trial for Safety and Immunogenicity of a Chikungunya Vaccine, VRC-CHKVLP059-00-VP, in Healthy Adults. NCT02562482.

2015. Available from: https://www.cochranelibrary.com/central/doi/10.1002/central/CN-01492587/full

[92] ClinicalTrials.gov. Trial of a Chikungunya Vaccine, PXVX0317 CHIKV-VLP, in Healthy Adults. NCT03483961. Epub ahead of print 2018. Available from: https://clinicaltrials.gov/ct2/show/NCT03483961

[93] Clinical. Safety and Immunogenicity of CHIKV VLP Vaccine PXVX0317 in Adults ≥65 Years. NCT05349617. Epub ahead of print 2022. Available from: https://clinicaltrials.gov/ct2/show/NCT05349617

[94] ClinicalTrials.gov. Phase II Study to Evaluate Safety and Immunogenicity of a Chikungunya Vaccine (MV-CHIK-202). NCT02861586. Epub ahead of print 2016. Available from: https://clinicaltrials.gov/ct2/show/NCT02861586

[95] ClinicalTrials.gov. Safety, Tolerability, and Immunogenicity of VAL-181388 in Healthy Subjects. NCT03325075. Epub ahead of print 2017. Available from: https://clinicaltrials.gov/ct2/show/NCT03325075

[96] ClinicalTrials.gov. Safety, Tolerability, Pharmacokinetics, and Pharmacodynamics of mRNA-1944 in Healthy Adults. NCT03829384. Epub ahead of print 2019. Available from: https://clinicaltrials.gov/ct2/show/NCT03829384

[97] US SEC. United States security and exchange commission reports. Epub ahead of print 2018. Available from: https://www.sec.gov/Archives/edgar/data/1682852/ 0001682852190000 09/moderna10-k12312018.htm

[98] Stapleford KA, Moratorio G, Henningsson R, et al. Whole-genome sequencing analysis from the chikungunya virus Caribbean outbreak reveals novel evolutionary genomic elements. PLoS Neglected Tropical Diseases. 2016;**10**:1-18

[99] Zakotnik S, Korva M, Knap N, et al. Complete coding sequence of a chikungunya virus strain imported into Slovenia from Thailand in late 2018. Microbiology Resource Announcements. 2019;**8**:1-3

[100] Redoni M, Yacoub S, Rivino L, et al. Dengue: Status of current and under-development vaccines. Reviews in Medical Virology. 2020;**30**:e2101

[101] Amorim JH, Birbrair A. Dengue vaccines: Where are we now and where we are going? The Lancet Infectious Diseases. 2022;**22**:756-757

[102] Deng SQ, Yang X, Wei Y, et al. A review on dengue vaccine development. Vaccine. 2020;**8**:1-13

[103] Pinheiro-Michelsen JR, da Souza RSO, IVR S, et al. Anti-dengue vaccines: From development to clinical trials. Frontiers in Immunology. 2020;**11**:1-18

[104] Rothe C, Boecken G, Rosenbusch D, et al. Travel vaccinations. Bundesgesundheitsblatt - Gesundheitsforsch - Gesundheitsschutz. 2020;**63**:74-84

[105] Richner JM, Jagger BW, Shan C, et al. Vaccine mediated protection against Zika virus-induced congenital disease. Cell. 2017;**170**:273-283

[106] Pardi N, Hogan MJ, Pelc RS, et al. Zika virus protection by a single low-dose nucleoside-modified mRNA vaccination. Nature. 2017;**543**:248-251

[107] ModernaTX Inc. Safety, Tolerability, and Immunogenicity of Zika Vaccine mRNA-1893 in

Healthy Flavivirus Seropositive and Seronegative Adults. NCT04064905. Epub ahead of print 2019. Available from: https://clinicaltrials.gov/ct2/show/NCT04064905

[108] ModernaTX Inc. A Study of Zika Vaccine mRNA-1893 in Adult Participants Living in Endemic and Non-Endemic Flavivirus Areas. NCT04917861. Epub ahead of print 2021. Available from: https://clinicaltrials.gov/ct2/show/results/NCT04917861

[109] Luisi K, Morabito KM, Burgomaster KE, et al. Development of a potent Zika virus vaccine using self-amplifying messenger RNA. Science Advances. 2020;**6**:1-10

[110] Erasmus JH, Khandhar AP, Guderian J, et al. A nanostructured lipid carrier for delivery of a replicating viral RNA provides single, low-dose protection against Zika. Molecular Therapy. 2018;**26**:2507-2522

[111] Armbruster N, Jasny E, Petsch B. Advances in rna vaccines for preventive indications: A case study of a vaccine against rabies. Vaccine. 2019;**7**:1-12

[112] Stokes A, Pion J, Binazon O, et al. Nonclinical safety assessment of repeated administration and biodistribution of a novel rabies self-amplifying mRNA vaccine in rats: Toxicity and biodistribution of rabies SAM vaccine. Regulatory Toxicology and Pharmacology. 2020;**113**:1-13

[113] Aldrich C, Leroux–Roels I, Huang KB, et al. Proof-of-concept of a low-dose unmodified mRNA-based rabies vaccine formulated with lipid nanoparticles in human volunteers: A phase 1 trial. Vaccine 2021;**39**:1310-1318

[114] Alberer M, Gnad-Vogt U, Hong HS, et al. Safety and immunogenicity of a mRNA rabies vaccine in healthy adults: An open-label, non-randomised, prospective, first-in-human phase 1 clinical trial. Lancet. 2017;**390**:1511-1520

[115] ClinicalTrials.gov. A Study to Evaluate the Safety and Immunogenicity of GlaxoSmithKline (GSK) Biologicals' Experimental Rabies Vaccine in Healthy Adults. NCT04062669. Epub ahead of print 2019. Available from: https://clinicaltrials.gov/ct2/show/NCT04062669

[116] Farman A, Lal Badshah S, Khan K, et al. Ebola, The negative stranded RNA virus. In: Some RNA Viruses. London UK: IntechOpen; 2021. Epub ahead of print 2021. DOI: 10.5772/intechopen.91776

[117] GISAID. Dataset Ebola. 2014. Available from: https://www.gisaid.org/epiflu-applications/influenza-genomic-epidemiology/ [Accessed: 2 July 2022]

[118] UCSC Genome Browser. UCSC Genome Browser on Ebola virus Sierra Leone 2014 (G3683/KM034562.1/eboVir3). 2014. Available from: https://genome.ucsc.edu/cgi- bin/hgTracks?db=eboVir3&lastVirtModeType=default&lastVirtModeExtraSt ate=&virtModeType=default&virtMode=0&nonVirtPosition=&position=KM0 34562v1%3A1-18957&hgsid=1402814645_u78A5PrvjdbW9kohP8KxU6awdcU6 [Accessed: 2 July 2022]

[119] Wang Y, Li J, Hu Y, et al. Ebola vaccines in clinical trial: The promising candidates. Human Vaccines & Immunotherapeutics. 2017;**13**:153-168

[120] Ishola D, Manno D, Afolabi MO, et al. Safety and long-term immunogenicity of the two-dose heterologous Ad26.ZEBOV and MVA-BN-filo Ebola vaccine regimen in adults in Sierra Leone: A combined open-label, non-randomised stage 1, and a

randomised, double-blind, controlled stage 2 trial. The Lancet Infectious Diseases. 2022;**22**:97-109

[121] Schwartz DA. Being Pregnant during the Kivu Ebola Virus Outbreak in DR Congo: The rVSV-ZEBOV Vaccine and Its Accessibility by Mothers and Infants during Humanitarian Crises and in Conflict Areas. Vaccines. 2020;**8**:1-18

[122] Hoff NA, Bratcher A, Daniel Kelly J, et al. Immunogenicity of rVSVΔG-ZEBOV-GP Ebola vaccination in exposed and potentially exposed persons in the Democratic Republic of the Congo. Proceedings of the National Academy of Sciences. PNAS. 2022;**119**:1-7

[123] ClinicalTrials.gov. Open-Label Study of INO-4212 With or Without INO-9012, Administered IM or ID Followed by Electroporation in Healthy Volunteers. NCT02464670. Available from: https://clinicaltrials.gov/ct2/show/NCT02464670

[124] ClinicalTrials.gov. INO-4201 as Booster in Healthy VSV-ZEBOV Vaccinees (Boost-EBOV). NCT04906629. Epub ahead of print 2021. Available from: https://clinicaltrials.gov/ct2/show/NCT04906629

[125] Meyer M, Huang E, Yuzhakov O, et al. Modified mRNA-Based Vaccines Elicit Robust Immune Responses and Protect Guinea Pigs From Ebola Virus Disease. Journal of Infectious Diseases. 2018;**217**:451-455

[126] Cu Y, Broderick K, Banerjee K, et al. Enhanced delivery and potency of self-amplifying mRNA vaccines by electroporation in situ. Vaccine. 2013;**1**:367-383

Chapter 3

Ribozymes as Therapeutic Agents against Infectious Diseases

Bao Chi Wong, Umama Shahid and Hock Siew Tan

Abstract

Ribozymes, also known as RNA enzymes, are catalytic RNA molecules capable of cleaving specific RNA sequences, leading to decreased expression of targeted genes. Recent studies suggest their role in cancer therapeutics, genetic diseases and retroviral infections. This book chapter will focus on ribozymes acting as therapeutic agents against infectious diseases caused by viral and bacterial pathogens. Firstly, we will introduce a brief history of ribozymes and a general overview of ribozymes and their characteristics. Next, different types of ribozymes will be explored regarding their targets and mechanisms of action. After that, ribozymes specific to viral and bacterial infections will be explored. We will briefly discuss the current status of ribozymes as therapeutic agents. Finally, the roadblock and challenges ribozymes face before being developed into therapeutic agents—such as their delivery and efficacy issues—will be discussed.

Keywords: ribozymes, therapeutic agent, antiviral, antibacterial, infectious diseases

1. Introduction

Proteins have always been the undefeated champions in most stories that any molecular biologist has to tell. A classic textbook elaborates extensively on these molecules, their structures, localisations and functions, followed by an essential section on enzymes. The Central Dogma of Molecular Biology states that deoxy-ribonucleic acid (DNA) precedes protein. DNA encodes important information, is converted into ribonucleic acid (RNA) and finally translated into the master molecule, protein [1]. So, in principle, proteins cannot exist without nucleic acids. However, the precursor here, i.e. DNA, is not even capable of replicating, much less forming a protein by itself, because it is found in a double-stranded form and hence is functionally inert. Therefore, DNA requires something capable of catalysing these reactions. Biologists have tried to explore the players involved in this phenomenon for years until a relatively recent discovery of catalytic RNAs by Thomas Cech and Sidney Altman proposed a possible explanation [2].

In 1978, Thomas Cech (University of Colorado) and his team decided to study RNA splicing, a considerably new field at the time. To explore RNA processing, they started working with a ciliated protozoan, *Tetrahymena thermophila*. Ribosomal RNA was chosen owing to its abundant amount in the selected system [3]. The 26S rRNA gene in *Tetrahymena* includes an intron of about 400 nucleotides, which must be removed before the gene product can localise and function as required. However, they observed a 9S RNA fragment (approximately 400 nucleotides) in all their phenol-based nuclear extractions, leading them to assume the possibility of protein contamination in the nuclear extracts, which was responsible for the splicing of this intron. Extreme efforts were made to remove/denature the protein that was thought to be either contaminant or strongly attached to the RNA molecules. The samples were subjected to high salt concentrations and exposed to high temperatures (both being something that a protein does not like), but splicing was observed, nonetheless. This result hinted that no protein could be present/responsible for the processing. However, this was not enough evidence. Kruger et al. described the cloning of the *Tetrahymena* rRNA gene in the *Escherichia coli* plasmid, followed by its *in vitro* transcription in their 1982 article [4]. The rRNA thus transcribed was also capable of excising the intron itself, proving that it was, in fact, a self-splicing molecule and did not require any protein for the processing. In the same year, Cech and his team released an article explaining the actual working of rRNA self-splicing where they showed that a GTP was required as a co-factor [5]. A detailed mechanism of self-splicing will be explained later in this chapter.

The discovery of self-splicing RNA molecules raised consciousness in the molecular biology world. Where one set of researchers dismissed it by calling the finding 'not a big deal', others started investigating the possibility of more reactions that were catalysed by RNA. Sidney Altman, Norman Pace and their respective teams studied ribonuclease P, an enzyme responsible for tRNA processing. Ribonuclease P is an interesting molecule since 80% of its content is RNA, and only 10% is protein. Initially, the RNA part of ribonuclease P was considered leftover contamination from protein purification with no significance. However, both teams demonstrated that reactions could occur without the protein section of ribonuclease P, proving that the RNA component catalysed the cleavage [6]. In 1989, Cech and Altman shared a Nobel prize in chemistry for demonstrating the catalytic activity of RNA. Many terms were coined for these special RNA molecules, now named Ribozymes (Ribonucleic acids that act as enzymes). Though not as common in vertebrates, RNA catalysis is now known to be widely spread amongst bacteria, viruses, some lower eukaryotes and even plants. One is also found in humans [7]. The naturally occurring ribozymes are reported to aid in reactions such as Ribosyl 2'-O mediated cleavage [8], RNA cleavage and ligation [9], DNA cleavage and ligation [10], etc. In addition, researchers worldwide are generating artificial ribozymes through combinatorial screening of random RNA sequences, which has increased the catalytic repertoire to an even larger range, including phosphorylation [11], acyl transfer reaction [12] and an amazing RNA polymerase ribozyme capable of polymerising complex RNA structures such as aptamers, ribozymes and even tRNA, amongst others [13].

2. General characteristics of ribozymes

Catalytic RNAs, like proteins, form a 3-D structure to be functionally sound for catalysis. Metal ions such as K^+ or Mg^{2+} are required for the proper folding of ribozymes to recompense for the high negative charge of the oligonucleotides [14]. Ribozymes typically contribute to self-targeted reactions (such as self-cleavage, self-splicing, ligation and template-directed polymerisation) except for one, i.e. RNase P (involved in the processing of tRNA) [15]. RNA has a limited range of chemical functionalities with just four similar nucleotides as building blocks. Despite this,

RNA can catalyse phosphoryl transfer reactions by about a million-fold, if not more [16]. Generally, naturally occurring ribozymes catalyse these reactions by attacking sugar 2′ or 3′-hydroxyl on a phosphodiester linkage. This nucleophilic attack involves activation of the nucleophile, stabilisation of an electronegative transition state and stabilisation of the leaving group.

Ribozymes can be categorised into two categories based on their size and whether a ribozyme uses its sugar -OH group to target the 3′ phosphodiester bond or requires an exogenous nucleophile [15]. The first group is the small ribozymes (approximately 35–155 nucleotides) that utilise 2′-hydroxyl of an adjacent nucleotide for the nucleophilic attack. The second group is the large ribozymes (approximately 200–3000 nucleotides) that attack using exogenous groups such as water, hydroxyl group from a mononucleotide or even a distantly located nucleotide from the same stretch [17]. Ribozymes perform phosphoryl transfer reactions using two main mechanisms, which are acid-base catalysis (seen in hammerhead, hairpin and *glmS* ribozymes) and metal-ion-assisted catalysis (seen in RNase P, group I, group II introns, HDV ribozymes) [17].

2.1 Small self-cleaving ribozymes

In general, small self-cleaving ribozymes act on the same strand, i.e. act in *cis* and hence, have a single catalytic turnover. These classes work on general acid-base catalysis. They use adjacent nucleobases or external co-factors as the general base or acid. The base takes a proton from the 2′-hydroxyl group, thereby increasing oxygen's nucleophilicity, which can then attack the nearby phosphorous. As a result, a transition state is formed. On the other hand, 5′-oxygen gets protonated by a general acid leading to the release of leaving group and thus the formation of 2′,3′-cyclic phosphate and a free 5′-hydroxyl group (**Figure 1**) [18]. Below are the different classes of small self-cleaving ribozymes.

With a size of about 40–50 nucleotides, the **hammerhead ribozyme** is, by far, the most extensively studied. Originally found in plant viroids and satellites, they are a widely spread class of self-cleaving RNAs known to catalyse the conversion

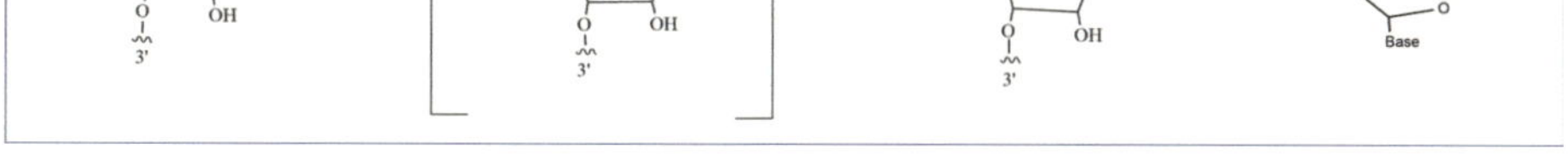

Figure 1.
Mechanism of catalysis in ribozymes: Ribozymes perform reversible nucleophilic reactions. (A) General Acid-Base catalysis. The general base (blue) deprotonates the 2′-hydroxyl in the cleavage reaction (or the 5′-hydroxyl in the reversed ligation reaction). The general acid (red) donates a proton to the 5′-oxyanion leaving group for cleavage (or the 2′oxyanion for ligation). A trigonal bipyramidal phosphorane is formed in the transition state (shown in the centre). B) RNA metalloenzymes. Large ribozymes, including RNase P and self-splicing introns, catalyse the phosphodiester bond breakdown via metal-ion catalysis. The figure is a representative group I intron where three metal ions bind to the transition state to bring about catalysis.

of their trimeric and dimeric forms into monomeric RNAs [19]. They are made up of three helical regions (Stem I, II, III), which are variable and a universally conserved junction sequence made up of three single strands (**Figure 2**) [20]. Hammerhead ribozymes cleave after an NUH [21] or NHH [22] triplet, where N can be any nucleotide, and H is any nucleotide except guanosine. They utilise N1 of G12 from stem II in their catalysis as a nucleophile. It forms a hydrogen bond with 2′ hydroxyl of C17 [23]. Some studies report that a divalent metal cation helps activate G12. Stabilisation of G8 occurs due to its base pairing with G3 [24]. Earlier, the 2′-hydroxyl group of G8 was thought to be the acid in this acid-base catalysis. However, a recent study reports that Mn^{2+}-bound water is the general acid during cleavage [25].

Hairpin ribozymes, like hammerhead ribozymes, are also found in plants' satellite viruses such as the tobacco ringspot (best studied), chicory yellow mottle and Arabis mosaic virus also catalyse the self-cleavage of multimeric RNA [26]. They comprise four stems that, when aligned, resemble a hairpin (**Figure 2**). A10 and G11 and A24 and C25 assemble as a ribose zipper and form a catalytic centre. The general base, in this case, is G8 (stem B), and A38 a (stem A) acts as a general acid, respectively. Rigorous *in vitro* selection of active mutants has shown that hairpin ribozymes prefer G at the +1 position of their cleavage site. N*GUY emerged as the best agreed-upon cleavage site, where N is any nucleotide, G is guanine, U is uracil and Y is any pyrimidine [27]. Later studies showed that substrates with G*GUN, G*GGR (R is any purine) and U*GUA could also be cleaved but with a considerably lower catalytic activity [28]. A crowded environment near the hairpin ribozymes increases their activity by stabilising the active conformation [29].

Hepatitis delta virus-like ribozymes are self-cleaving ribozymes present in the genomic strand and the complementary/anti-genomic strand found in Hepatitis delta virus (HDV) (a single-stranded RNA virus that infects mammalian hepatocytes) [30]. These ribozymes also catalyse a transesterification reaction through a nucleophilic attack by a 2′ hydroxyl on the adjacent phosphate and result in the formation of a 2′–3′ cyclic phosphates and the release of 5′ hydroxyls. Their structure consists of five paired regions of helices, which, when coaxially aligned, are stacked over each other (P1 over P1.1 and P4; P2 over P3). Single-stranded joining strands link these helices. Crystallography reveals that they assume an extremely stable structure resembling a double pseudoknot. HDV-like ribozymes cleave at the first guanosine residue at the base of the P1 helix [31].

The **glucosamine-6-phosphate synthase (*glmS*) ribozyme** is found in several Gram-positive bacteria in the 5' UTR region of the *glmS* gene [32]. It regulates the expression of glutamine-fructose-6-phosphate transaminase and is the only known ribozyme which requires glucosamine-6-phosphate (GlcN6P) as a co-factor [33]. The *glmS* ribozyme comprises three parallel helices stacking each other (P1 on P3.1, P4 on P4.1 and P2.1). It also forms a core resembling a double pseudoknot. P3 and P4 are not essential for catalysis. However, they provide structural stability and enhance the activity of ribozymes. The P2.2 forms the binding site for GlcN6P, and the correct folding of P2.2 brings the ribozyme into active conformation [34]. A co-factor is required for the protonation of the 5′ oxygen leaving group, activation of the 2′-oxygen nucleophile and charge stabilisation [35].

Largest nucleolytic RNA with a length of ~150 nucleotides, the **Varkud Satellite (VS) ribozymes** are found in certain strains of Neurospora and help in the replication of single-stranded RNA [15]. VS ribozymes comprise seven helices (1–7), forming a three-way junction (2-3-6, 3-4- and 1-7-2). The inner loops of stem 1 act as their

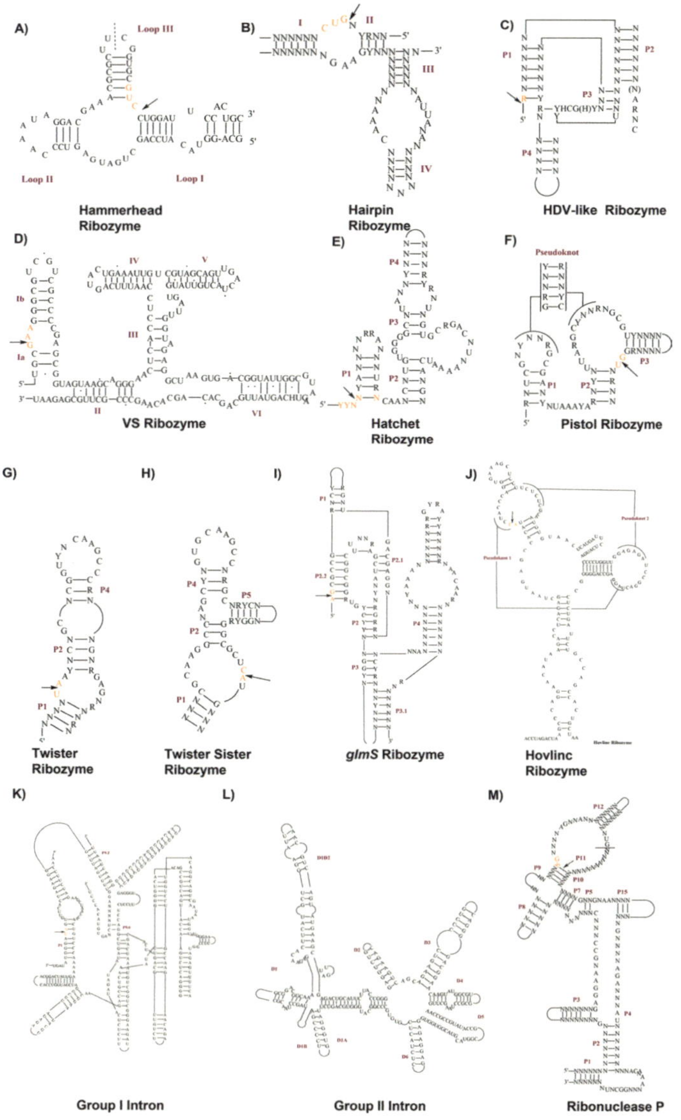

Figure 2.
Consensus secondary structures ribozymes. A, U, G and C represent adenine, uracil, guanine and cytosine. N represents any nucleotide. R stands for any purine and Y for any pyrimidine. The black arrows show the cleavage site, orange-coded nucleotides represent conserved bases near the cleavage sites, and the solid line shows a variable stretch of nucleotides.

cleavage site, while stems 6 and 1 harbour the catalytic centre [36]. A kissing loop forms between GUC in stem 1 and GAC in stem 5 to form an active site, bringing the cleavage site to the catalytic centre. The residues A756 and G638 act as the general acid and base, respectively. Additionally, Mg^{2+} is reported to interact with scissile phosphate and activate G638 [37].

Hatchet ribozymes are one of the bioinformatically revealed ribozymes, and very little is known about them. They comprise four stems (P1–P4). P1 and P2 are linked with highly conserved residues, whereas internal loops (L2 and L3) connect the other three stems [38]. X-ray crystallography reveals that they appear as pseudo symmetrical RNA and form long-range interactions of conserved residues near scissile phosphate. The cleavage site is located at the 5′ end of the P1 stem. N7 of G31 acts as the general base to deprotonate the 2′-OH of C (−1) for nucleophilic attack. In addition, Mg^{2+} is required for proper folding and catalysis [39].

Twister ribozymes are widely spread among many species of bacteria and eukaryotes [40]. They are made up of five stems (P1–P5) and internal loops held together by two pseudoknots. Twister ribozymes cleave folding-dependently, where central pseudoknot opens and closes at variable Mg^{2+} concentration [41]. These cations help position the phosphate oxygen at the U-A cleavage site and stabilise the transition stage to form an intermediate. Guanine is a conserved residue at the cleavage site. It acts as a general base in the general acid-base catalysis, whereas an adenine residue plays as the general acid. The active site comprises at least 10 conserved nucleotides, harbouring scissile phosphate between A and U joining P1 [42].

Twister sister ribozymes are highly similar to twister ribozymes in sequence and secondary structure. The only difference is that they do not have a double pseudoknot interaction. Long-range interactions that bring conserved nucleotides closer to the core are mediated by Mg^{2+} cations [43]. C62 and A63 flank the cleavage site on the internal loop between P1 and P2. Hydrogen bonds (N1H of G5, inner-sphere water of Mg^{2+} and phosphate oxygen) keep the scissile phosphate in its place [44]. The substrate specificity of these ribozymes has not been studied in detail yet.

Pistol ribozymes were discovered bioinformatically through comparative genomic analysis to search hammerhead and twister ribozymes-related sequences. Pistol ribozymes consist of three helical stems (P1–P3) connected by three loops (loops 1–3) and one pseudoknot. P1 and pseudoknot form a stacked structure [45]. N1 of G40 acts as a general base, and A32 acts as a general acid. Crystallography shows that Mg^{2+} cations have a significant role in catalysis. All information on this ribozyme is limited; some studies suggest that residues at positions 32 and 40 might affect the substrate specificity [46].

Hovlinc ribozymes are a recently discovered class of ribozymes that came up in a genome-wide search of human catalytic RNAs [47]. Although very little is known about hovlinc ribozymes, structure analysis shows that their catalytic core comprises two stem loops and two pseudoknots. They are pH-dependent and require divalent cations where their activity was shown to be highest in the presence of Mn^{2+} ($Mn^{2+} > Mg^{2+} > Ca^{2+}$) [48]. Further studies will be required to properly reveal its characteristic folding, cleavage site, catalytic centre and functioning.

2.2 Large ribozymes

These are often called ‘true catalysts’ because they can act on a substrate in a *trans* manner and thus have a catalytic turnover. In contrast to the small self-cleaving ribozymes, large catalytic RNAs act as metalloenzymes [7]. Metal ions are usually found in the active sites of these ribozymes and form inner-sphere complexes with oxygen atoms of the RNA (**Figure 1**).

Introns are intervening noncoding regions between a gene’s exon (coding regions). When a gene is transcribed, the pre-RNA thus formed undergoes removal, i.e. splicing all the introns to obtain mature RNA [49]. Naturally found in bacteria and bacteriophages, nuclear rRNA genes and chloroplast DNA, **Group I introns** are self-splicing in nature and can excise themselves without a protein enzyme [50]. These can migrate and insert themselves at different positions of the host genome, thus acting as mobile genetic elements [51]. Although widespread, the group I ribozymes have very less sequence similarity. However, they all can fold into a conserved secondary structure with 10 paired segments (P1–P10). The catalytic core comprises P3, P4, P6 and P7 [9]. The intron is spliced from the pre-RNA by a two-step transesterification reaction. First, 3′ hydroxyl makes a nucleophilic attack on a guanosine co-factor at the 5′ splice site. The exon-intron phosphodiester bond is cleaved, and guanosine forms a 3′,5′-phosphodiester bond at the 5′ ends of the intron. Finally, a nucleophilic attack of now free 3′ hydroxyl of the 5′ at the 3′ splice site to form the ligated exons results in the release of an intron with the nonencoded guanosine. The intron is circularised by making a nucleophilic attack with its highly conserved 3′ terminal guanosine at a phosphodiester bond of C-15 or C-19. Each step is fully reversible and follows the SN2 reaction mechanism [52].

The self-splicing **group II introns** are widespread amongst the mRNA, tRNA and rRNA genes of plant and fungal mitochondria and chloroplasts (including algae and protists) [51]. The secondary structure of Group II introns was initially revealed via computational modelling and phylogenetic comparisons. They are composed of six helices (I–VI) radiating from a centrally located wheel [53]. Out of the six helical domains present, only I and V are crucial for their activity. Domain V, the most variable region, harbours the active site. A conserved Adenosine residue is present in the domain, which initiates the splicing reaction. 2′-Hydroxyl of adenosine performs the nucleophilic attack and forms a structure known as a lariat, which contains 3′–5′ and 2′–5′ phosphodiester bonds at the adenosine branch site. Following this, free 3′-hydroxyl of 5′ exon makes a nucleophilic attack at the 3′ splice site resulting in ligated exons and spliced out intron (as a lariat). Though not common, a nucleophilic attack may sometimes be initiated by water, resulting in a linear intron [54].

RNase P is a widespread enzyme processing tRNA precursors [55]. It is known to exist in a ribonucleoprotein complex consisting of about 350–400 nucleotide long RNA stretch and about 14kDa of small protein subunit [56]. Though protein moiety is important for catalysis *in vivo*, the RNA component is enough *in vitro*. The reaction occurs at a high salt concentration, and protein was assumed to promote RNA enzyme and substrate interaction. However, studies have shown that the protein component of RNase P plays a significant role in site specificity and turnover [57]. No high sequence conservation is observed in RNase P across different organisms. However, they all can fold into a similar secondary structure [56]. RNase P from *E. coli* M1 RNA consists of 18 paired helices, but RNase P from *Bacillus subtilis* lacks P6, P13, P14, P16 and P17 but contains a few extra helices (P5.1, P10.1, P15.1 and P19). Despite these differences, comparative analyses of RNase P secondary structure have deduced a catalytic core composed of P1–P5, P7–12 and P15. This ribozyme uses water to make a nucleophilic attack [58].

In eukaryotic cells, intron removal occurs through a ribonucleoprotein complex called **spliceosomes**. These complexes are not preformed; five RNAs and about 100 proteins assemble directly into a spliceosome on their substrate [59]. Splicing events can be divided into four main reaction steps: assembly, activation, catalysis and disassembly [60, 61]. The catalytic centre of spliceosomes highly resembles Group II introns, and even the splicing mechanism is quite like the latter [62].

The **ribosome** is a protein translating machinery formed by 30S and 50S subunits in bacteria and 40S and 60S subunits in eukaryotes, respectively [63]. The larger subunit contains the peptidyl transferase centre (PTC), which forms peptides by joining amino acids. X-ray crystallography and electron microscopy have elucidated two main reactions involved in protein synthesis: aminolysis to form peptide bonds and peptidyl hydrolysis to release protein after synthesis. The catalysis does not occur via nucleobase-mediated catalysis, rather is mediated by 2′-hydroxyl of tRNA [64]. Both these reactions occur in the PTC, known to be made completely of RNA [65].

3. Ribozymes as antiviral and antibacterial infection alternatives

The potential of ribozymes as therapeutic agents has been explored from other perspectives, including cancer and inherited diseases. Ribozymes downregulate the expression of the target gene(s) through the cleavage of mRNA transcripts. If the expression of a gene could lead to pathogenesis, then the downregulation of that gene expression via ribozymes can be performed as a therapeutic option. Previous studies have selected a few important genes responsible for viral replication as targets. By decreasing the viral replication, the application of ribozymes will inevitably treat the viral infection.

Multiple viruses have been used as targets in antiviral ribozyme research, including the human immunodeficiency virus (HIV), herpes simplex virus (HSV) and human cytomegalovirus. Different types of ribozymes were used, demonstrating their potential to be used as therapeutic agents in both *in vitro* and *in vivo* conditions (**Table 1**). There are different strategies for studying the efficiency of antiviral ribozymes. If a target gene is shortlisted and the cleavage site is determined, the ribozyme can be designed rationally. If the cleavage site is undetermined, the potential target cleavage site can be screened to discover any region exposed to the ribozyme for easy binding. Another method is to use a library of ribozymes to find any ribozymes with

Target	Ribozyme	Design	Delivery	References
Herpes simplex virus (HSV)				
Thymidine kinase	RNase P	*In vitro* selection	Endogenous—Retrovirus	[66]
Infected-cell polypeptide 4 (ICP4)	RNase P (M1GS)	*In vitro* selection	Endogenous—Retrovirus	[67]
Latency-associated transcript (LAT)	Hammerhead	Rational design	Endogenous—Adenovirus	[68]
Human cytomegalovirus				
Capsid assembly protein (AP) and protease (PR)	RNase P (M1GS)	Rational design	Endogenous—Retrovirus	[69]
Assembly protein (mAP) and M80	RNase P (M1GS)	Rational design	Endogenous—Retrovirus (*in vitro*); hydrodynamic transfection (murine)	[70]
M80.5 and protease	RNase P (M1GS)	Rational design	Endogenous—Salmonella	[71]
Immediate early proteins 1 and 2	RNase P	Screening of target sites	Endogenous—Retrovirus	[72]
Assemblin (AS)	RNase P (M1GS)	*In vitro* selection	Endogenous—Retrovirus (*in vitro*); hydrodynamic transfection (murine)	[73]

Target	Ribozyme	Design	Delivery	References
Human immunodeficiency virus 1 (HIV-1)				
Vpr and tat region	Hammerhead	Rational design	Endogenous—Retrovirus	[74]
Glycoprotein (gp41)	Hammerhead	Rational design	Exogenous	[75]
Tat region	RNase P	*In vitro* selection	Endogenous—Retrovirus	[76]
Glycoprotein (gp41)	Hammerhead	Rational design	Endogenous—Plasmid	[77]
Influenza A virus				
Conserved regions of Influenza A virus mRNA	Hepatitis delta virus ribozyme	Rational design	Endogenous—Plasmid	[78]
Conserved RNA secondary structure motifs	Hammerhead	Rational design	Endogenous—Plasmid	[79]
Sindbis virus				
Within the 26S subgenomic RNA	Hairpin	Rational design	Endogenous—Plasmid	[80]
Genomic RNA	Hairpin	Screening of target sites	Endogenous—Plasmid	[81]
Chikungunya virus				
Conserved genomic sequences among 100 strains	Hammerhead	Rational design	Endogenous—Retrovirus (*in vitro*); *piggyBac* vector (mosquito)	[82]
Hepatitis C virus				
5′ UTR of HCV genome	M1GS ribozyme	Rational design	Exogenous	[83]
SARS virus and mouse hepatitis virus (MHV)				
SARS and MHV consensus sequences	Chimeric DNA-RNA hammerhead	Rational design	Exogenous	[84]

Table 1.
Examples of antiviral ribozymes.

high binding or cleavage activity towards the target virus. Finally, two main delivery methods exist for introducing ribozymes into the system. While some studies propose the potential of ribozymes as therapeutic agents for viral infections, there is still a distinct lack of ribozymes that successfully passed their pre-clinical or clinical trials.

To our best knowledge, there are currently no studies on using ribozymes to cleave specific target genes in bacteria to treat bacterial infections. Instead, Felletti et al. [85] successfully cleaved the bacterial 3′-untranslated region (UTR) using twister ribozymes, affecting the expression of the gene downstream. By designing the ribozymes specific to the 3′-UTR of essential bacterial genes, these ribozymes have potential as antibacterial agents.

4. Current status of ribozymes

As of 2022, only four clinical trials are registered on ClinicalTrials.gov for using ribozymes as therapeutic agents (**Table 2**). Among these four, three clinical trials are targeted towards human immunodeficiency virus (HIV), while the other ribozyme is targeted towards kidney cancer.

Two clinical trials were conducted for OZ1, a ribozyme designed to target the overlapping region between two essential genes. The multifunctional viral protein R (vpr) is involved in host infection, immune system evasion and infection persistence [86]. The tat protein is also involved in viral replication, enhancing the efficiency of viral expression [87]. The ribozyme OZ1 is a hammerhead ribozyme encoded within a Moloney murine leukaemia gammaretroviral vector LNL6 [74]. By cleaving the overlapping region in the *vpr* and *tat* gene, the ribozyme could inhibit the replication of HIV-1. A phase I clinical trial was conducted by delivering the OZ1 ribozyme through a retroviral vector to the mature CD34+ hematopoietic cells [74]. It was determined that the gene expression of ribozyme was detected within the patients, demonstrating that the ribozyme OZ1 can be maintained. Another Phase I study was done using a similar delivery vector to CD4+ T lymphocytes, demonstrating similar results whereby the cells can express the ribozyme long term [88]. A Phase II clinical trial (NCT00074997) was conducted with OZ1 ribozymes targeting the CD34+ hematopoietic cells. They did not achieve their primary efficacy endpoint as the mean

Title of clinical trial	Ribozyme	Target gene	Disease	NCT number	Time
An Efficacy and Safety Study of Autologous Cluster of Differentiation 34 (CD34+) Hematopoietic Progenitor Cells Transduced With Placebo or an Anti-Human Immunodeficiency Virus Type 1 (HIV-1) Ribozyme (OZ1) in Participants With HIV-1 Infection	OZ1	vpr/tat	HIV-1	NCT00074997	2002–2008
Long Term Follow-Up Study of Human Immunodeficiency Virus Type 1 (HIV-1) Positive Patients Who Have Received OZ1 Gene Therapy as Part of a Clinical Trial	OZ1	vpr/tat	HIV-1	NCT01177059	2004–2017
Gene Therapy in HIV-Positive Patients With Non-Hodgkin's Lymphoma	L-TR / Tat-neo	Tat, Rev mRNA	Non-Hodgkin lymphoma, HIV infections	NCT00002221	2001 – N/A
RPI.4610 in Treating Patients With Metastatic Kidney Cancer	ANGIOZYME	VEGF-1	Kidney cancer	NCT00021021	2001–2004

Table 2.
Clinical trials of ribozymes registered on ClinicalTrials.gov. All trials were completed in phase 2 trials.

plasma HIV-1 viral load difference was lower but not significantly different from the placebo. However, no serious adverse events were linked to OZ1 gene transfer, indicating that using the retroviral vector to perform this gene therapy is safe, albeit with low efficacy. A second Phase II clinical trial (NCT01177059) was performed with the same group of patients from the previous trials to investigate the long-term effect of the ribozymes. There was no serious adverse effect on the participants due to the treatment. The OZ1 and the retroviral vector LNL6 marking analysis showed that they were only detected in a few participants. Unfortunately, there are no further studies on this ribozyme, perhaps due to its low efficiency in the human system.

Another Phase II clinical trial (NCT00002221) also investigated the usage of ribozymes against HIV. In this trial, a retrovirus containing two ribozyme sequences named L-TR/Tat-neo that target the tat and rev region of the virus RNA was used. Like the tat protein, the rev protein is also essential for viral replication [89]. The ribozymes were delivered to the participants of the clinical trials through *ex vivo* retroviral modified CD34+ stem cells. However, no results have been provided for this clinical trial.

Finally, RPI.4610 (ANGIOZYME), a ribozyme that targets vascular endothelial growth factor receptor 1 (VEGF1) was used to treat patients with metastatic kidney cancer. VEGF is an angiogenesis-promoting molecule, and when its preRNA is cleaved, it can inhibit angiogenesis and tumour growth [90–92]. Clinical trials with ANGIOZYME have demonstrated that it is well tolerated. However, due to its lack of efficacy, this drug could not proceed with further development [93].

5. The roadblock to commercialisation

While ribozymes have the potential to be one of the alternatives to treat infectious diseases, it cannot be denied that there are still multiple roadblocks before they can be developed as marketable drugs. Like other nucleic-acid therapeutics, ribozymes' challenges include selecting the appropriate ribozyme type and target mRNA sequence, delivery to the target site, efficiency *in vivo* and potential side effects as therapeutic drugs.

5.1 Selection of target and ribozymes

There is a wide variety of genes to choose from within the target pathogen, be it virus or bacteria, which can be used as a ribozyme target. The selection of these targets would thus depend on the aim of the ribozyme. An antiviral ribozyme may target the mRNA of genes important for viral replication, while an antibacterial ribozyme to decrease antibiotic resistance may target antimicrobial resistance genes (AMR) instead. More importantly, the cleavage site within the mRNA transcript must be carefully determined for the best cleavage efficiency. Designing sequence-specific ribozymes can be done through rational design or by *in vitro* selection.

To design a ribozyme that targets a specific gene, it needs a target-specific sequence that leads the ribozyme to the target mRNA transcript and cleaves it. Different ribozymes have different target cleavage sites due to their structural variety. For instance, hammerhead ribozymes have an NUH or NHH sequence specificity. In comparison, hairpin ribozymes catalyse site-specific reversible cleavage on the 5' side of a GUC triplet [94]. Another criterion to consider is the accessibility of the cleavage site to the ribozymes. RNAs can fold to specific three-dimensional structures; multiple methods exist to study these structures [95]. One of them is the usage of dimethyl sulfate (DMS), a chemical that can covalently modify both purines and pyrimidines that are accessible [96, 97]. Through DMS probing and footprinting, it is possible to detect the RNA secondary and even tertiary structure, determine the potential region most accessible to DMS modification and presumably ribozyme binding.

On the other hand, Zhang et al. used a random pool of ribozymes to find accessible target sites [81]. As we progress into the post-genomic era, some may look towards in-silico analysis and bioinformatics to determine the best cleavage site, shortlisting a few for wet lab validation. RiboSoft [98] and RiboSubstrates [99] are some web applications that allow a comprehensive ribozyme design. Unfortunately, these two websites are not maintained. RNAiFold is another web server used to design a hammerhead ribozyme through computational design with experimental validation, showing that this method can be used for synthetic ribozymes [100].

Other than rational design, another method to obtain specific and efficient ribozymes is through an *in vitro* selection process using a ribozyme library [101]. Multiple studies have used this process to identify ribozymes with high cleavage efficiency. A putative self-cleaving hairpin ribozyme library was used whereby ribozymes that successfully bind and cleave a target sequence were identified [102]. Not only does this method allows the identification of effective target sites within the target mRNA, but it can also identify the most efficient ribozyme for a particular target site. The in vitro selection was used by Maghami et al. [103] to identify efficient trans-acting adenylyl transferase ribozymes that can label specific RNA sites. The ribozymes developed can be modified to target other RNA sequences by changing the sequence-specific region of the ribozymes. This method can be modified to different types of ribozymes and towards different targets.

Finally, it is worth noting that while the discovery of ribozymes is not recent, there is still undiscovered land in this field. Firstly, ribozyme variants may provide higher efficiency in their catalytic activity, which can be discovered through *in vitro* selection from a random pool of ribozymes. Deep sequencing of a ribozyme library [104] or a high-throughput analysis [105] can help elucidate novel ribozymes and their properties. Secondly, new types of ribozymes are continually being discovered and studied. A new RNA polymerase ribozyme discovered can also act as a reverse transcriptase enzyme [106]. In contrast, a type of novel ribozyme called hatchet ribozyme was reported in 2019 [38], while a pseudoknot-type hammerhead ribozyme was studied in 2020 [19]. These discoveries demonstrate that new ribozymes with improved potential still continuously emerge in recent times.

5.2 Stability and delivery of ribozymes

Like most nucleic acids, Ribozymes are vulnerable to nuclease attacks by the host cells. An unmodified ribozyme would be rapidly degraded and would not be effective when exposed to nuclease-rich fluids and tissues. Additionally, some ribozymes require co-enzymes or a certain concentration of metal ions for sufficient stability and efficiency. For example, the *glmS* ribozyme-riboswitch requires the presence of the intracellular small molecule co-enzyme GlcN6P for effective catalysis [107]. On the other hand, divalent metal ions, such as magnesium ions, are generally required by ribozymes to form a tertiary structure or catalytic activity [108]. Certain modifications or delivery vectors are needed to ensure their efficiency *in vitro* and *in vivo*.

Ribozymes can be modified to improve their stability and resistance towards nucleases. Some modifications include using locked nucleic acids (LNAs) [109], cholesterol [83], nanoparticles [110], or low-molecular-weight polyethyleneimine [111]. Modifications to the ribozyme tertiary structure or interactions can improve their stability. For instance, a tertiary interaction between a GAAA tetraloop and a tetraloop receptor within a hammerhead ribozyme showed higher activity even under low magnesium conditions [75]. Another method of modification is to simply conduct an *in vitro* selection to determine which variants of ribozymes can remain effective. An RNase P ribozyme from *in vitro* selection showed a higher cleavage efficiency than the wild-type ribozyme. This variant was used towards the thymine kinase [66] and major transcription activator ICP4 [67] or the herpes simplex virus, as well as the assembly (AS) of murine cytomegalovirus [73]. A coenzyme-independent variant of *glmS* ribozyme was also successfully isolated through *in vitro* selection [112]. This variant contains the wild-type structure that can catalyse the cleaving reactions effectively with the presence of divalent cations alone. These studies demonstrate that it is feasible to develop variants of known ribozymes and modify their requirements for co-enzymes or increase their efficiency.

There are two ways to deliver the ribozymes into the cells: exogenous delivery (as preformed ribozymes) or endogenous delivery (as ribozyme genes). The preformed ribozymes can be delivered through electroporation or lipofection for exogenous delivery. A ribozyme stabilised by GAAA tetraloop and its receptor motif was transfected into human HeLa cells using Lipofectamine 2000 and showed effective target gene silencing [75]. A chimeric DNA-RNA hammerhead ribozyme was transfected using a polyethylenimine reagent into the cells [84]. Due to the vulnerability of ribozymes within the biological system, exogenous delivery relies on modifications that improve the stability of ribozymes. Other studies utilise endogenous delivery. In endogenous delivery, the ribozymes are introduced through ribozyme genes carried within plasmids or expression vectors. These plasmids can then be introduced through transfection to the cells, allowing the cells to express the ribozyme within the cytoplasm. The ribozymes can then catalyse the intended cleavage reaction within the cells [80, 81]. Besides plasmids, the ribozyme genes can be inserted in retroviral-derived or adeno-associated viral-derived vectors (refer to **Table 1**: Delivery). While unsuccessful, the clinical trials of multiple ribozymes using Moloney murine leukaemia virus retroviral vector LNL6 demonstrated its feasibility as delivery agents of ribozymes [113]. Endogenous delivery also benefits from modifications aiming to improve ribozyme stability. Peng et al. used a novel scaffold RNA to stabilise the ribozyme structure, improving its catalytic activities [114]. However, modifications performed on the ribozymes require further investigation. Czapik et al. showed that modifications such as adding a hairpin motif to the hammerhead ribozyme decreased their catalytic activity compared with the unmodified ribozymes [79].

The delivery methods of ribozymes are not limited to these traditional methods. Rouge *et al.* successfully transfected ribozymes into cancer cells without auxiliary transfection agents using the spherical nucleic acid (SNA) architecture to stabilise the ribozymes [110]. The ribozyme, targeted towards a gene involved in chemotherapeutic resistance of solid tumours, increased the sensitisation of the cancer cells towards therapy-mediated apoptosis. On the other hand, an attenuated strain of Salmonella that contains the expression vector encoding the ribozymes was used to deliver these ribozymes to mice [71]. The success of Salmonella-mediated oral delivery of the ribozymes introduced an alternative delivery method other than those mentioned before.

5.3 The efficiency of ribozymes under in vivo conditions

It is easily shown that they can cleave their target mRNA transcripts *in vitro* through the direct cleavage of RNAs or *in vitro* studies. However, it is not as simple to translate these data from *in vitro* conditions to *in vivo*. Multiple studies have used animal models to prove the potential therapeutic use of ribozymes, and they have successfully demonstrated that in models such as rats and rabbits. Nevertheless, there are still some challenges before the ribozymes can be used in the human body.

Ribozymes, like all enzymes, also require co-factors for their optimal function. One crucial co-factor is the divalent ions, such as magnesium ions. Mainly, these ions are required for the ribozymes to achieve the correct folding of the active site and their tertiary structures [108]. However, the requirements differ between ribozymes. For instance, magnesium is essential for the catalysis activity of hammerhead ribozymes, but hairpin ribozymes do not require magnesium [77, 115].

Further research into the effects of ion concentration on the catalytic core or structure of the ribozymes allowed specific modifications to be made. A section of the ribozyme responsible for substrate-binding and tertiary stabilisation functions can be separated into discrete structural segments to ensure that trans-cleaving hammerhead ribozymes can be used in intracellular applications [116]. This separation provided the resulting ribozymes with an efficient catalytic activity at lower magnesium ion concentration. Additionally, with careful selection, ribozymes may be evolved to require a lower concentration of metal ions for their efficient activity *in vitro* and *in vivo* [117].

Finally, the efficiency of the ribozymes to cleave their targets within the *in vivo* system is also a key to the success of ribozymes as antiviral or antibacterial therapeutic agents. As mentioned previously, the ribozyme ANGIOZYME, while showing promising results in pre-clinical trial studies, did not manage to proceed further than Phase 2 clinical trials due to their lack of efficiency in the patients [93]. Other studies have also highlighted the difficulty in translating the efficiency of ribozymes from *in vitro* to *in vivo*. Due to their rapid degradation during *in vivo* conditions decreasing their concentration within the system, it was proposed that ribozymes are more suitable for acute diseases and not chronic diseases [84]. There were also significant differences in the ribozyme efficiency in recognising and cleaving the target sequences when comparing *in vitro* and *in vivo* cells [77]. Due to these challenges, ribozymes' development as therapeutic agents, in general, has slowed down in the past years. More research must be conducted to improve the feasibility of ribozymes in the *in vivo* system by focusing on their stability and efficiency to bring ribozymes back to the table.

6. Conclusion

Ribozymes are catalytic RNAs that can catalyse reactions similarly to protein enzymes. There is a wide variety of ribozymes classes with different characteristics and structures, and even now, novel ribozymes are being discovered through research. Ribozymes have the potential to be used as therapeutic agents for infectious diseases. While there is a lack of actual ribozymes for antibacterial purposes, multiple ribozymes are tested to successfully target viruses such as human immunodeficiency virus (HIV), human cytomegalovirus and herpes simplex virus. Unfortunately, their uses have not been translated into real-world applications, mostly due to their vulnerability to nucleases in the biological system and the difficulty in translating their efficiency from the *in vitro* system to the *in vivo* system. However, progress has been made in improving their stability and delivery, and it is hoped that with more research, ribozymes can be the next therapeutic agent used for infectious diseases.

Acknowledgements

School of Science, Monash University Malaysia.

Conflict of interest

The authors do not have any conflict of interest.

Author details

Bao Chi Wong, Umama Shahid and Hock Siew Tan*
Monash University Malaysia, Selangor, Malaysia

*Address all correspondence to: tan.hocksiew@monash.edu

References

[1] Crick F. Central dogma of molecular biology. Nature. 1970;**227**(5258):561-563

[2] Gilbert W. Origin of life: The RNA world. Nature. 1986;**319**(6055):618

[3] Zaug AJ, Cech TR. The intervening sequence RNA of Tetrahymena is an enzyme. Science. 1986;**231**(4737):470-475

[4] Kruger K, Grabowski PJ, Zaug AJ, Sands J, Gottschling DE, Cech TR. Self-splicing RNA: Autoexcision and autocyclisation of the ribosomal RNA intervening sequence of Tetrahymena. Cell. 1982;**31**(1):147-157

[5] Zaug AJ, Cech TR. The intervening sequence excised from the ribosomal RNA precursor of Tetrahymena contains a 5-terminal guanosine residue not encoded by the DNA. Nucleic Acids Research. 1982;**10**(9):2823-2838

[6] Guerrier-Takada C, Gardiner K, Marsh T, Pace N, Altman S. The RNA moiety of ribonuclease P is the catalytic subunit of the enzyme. Cell. 1983;**35**(3 Pt 2):849-857

[7] Fedor MJ, Williamson JR. The catalytic diversity of RNAs. Nature Reviews. Molecular Cell Biology. 2005;**6**(5):399-412

[8] Burgin AB, Gonzalez C, Matulic-AdamicJ,KarpeiskyAM,UsmanN, McSwiggen JA, et al. Chemically modified hammerhead ribozymes with improved catalytic rates. Biochemistry. 1996;**35**(45):14090-14097

[9] Cech TR, Herschlag D. Group I ribozymes: Substrate recognition, catalytic strategies, and comparative mechanistic analysis. In: Eckstein F, DMJ L, editors. Catalytic RNA. Berlin, Heidelberg: Springer Berlin Heidelberg; 1997. pp. 1-17

[10] Tsang J, Joyce GF. Specialisation of the DNA-cleaving activity of a group I ribozyme through in vitro evolution. Journal of Molecular Biology. 1996;**262**(1):31-42

[11] Lorsch JR, Szostak JW. Kinetic and thermodynamic characterisation of the reaction catalysed by a polynucleotide kinase ribozyme. Biochemistry. 1995;**34**(46):15315-15327

[12] Lohse PA, Szostak JW. Ribozyme-catalysed amino-acid transfer reactions. Nature. 1996;**381**(6581):442-444

[13] Ekland EH, Bartel DP. RNA-catalysed RNA polymerisation using nucleoside triphosphates. Nature. 1996;**383**(6596):192

[14] Pyle AM. Role of metal ions in ribozymes. Metal Ions in Biological Systems. 1996;**32**:479-520

[15] Tanner NK. Ribozymes: The characteristics and properties of catalytic RNAs. FEMS Microbiology Reviews. 1999;**23**(3):257-275

[16] Wilson TJ, Lilley DMJ. The potential versatility of RNA catalysis. WIREs RNA. 2021;**12**(5):e1651

[17] Lilley DM. Mechanisms of RNA catalysis. Philosophical Transactions of the Royal Society of London. Series B, Biological Sciences. 2011;**366**(1580):2910-2917

[18] Ren A, Micura R, Patel DJ. Structure-based mechanistic insights into catalysis by small self-cleaving ribozymes.

Current Opinion in Chemical Biology. 2017;**41**:71-83

[19] Yamada M, Tanaka Y. Structure-activity relationship of pseudoknot-type hammerhead ribozyme reveals key structural elements for enhanced catalytic activity(†). Nucleosides, Nucleotides & Nucleic Acids. 2020;**39**(1-3):245-257

[20] McKay DB. Structure and function of the hammerhead ribozyme: An unfinished story. RNA. 1996;**2**(5):395-403

[21] Birikh KR, Heaton PA, Eckstein F. The structure, function and application of the hammerhead ribozyme. European Journal of Biochemistry. 1997;**245**(1):1-16

[22] Kore AR, Vaish NK, Kutzke U, Eckstein F. Sequence specificity of the hammerhead ribozyme revisited; the NHH rule. Nucleic Acids Research. 1998;**26**(18):4116-4120

[23] Wedekind JE, Mckay DB. Crystallographic structures of the hammerhead ribozyme: Relationship to Ribozyme Folding and Catalysis. Annual Review of Biophysics and Biomolecular Structure. 1998;**27**(1):475-502

[24] Lee TS, Silva López C, Giambasu GM, Martick M, Scott WG, York DM. Role of Mg2+ in hammerhead ribozyme catalysis from molecular simulation. Journal of the American Chemical Society. 2008;**130**(10):3053-3064

[25] Naghdi MR, Boutet E, Mucha C, Ouellet J, Perreault J. Single mutation in hammerhead ribozyme favors cleavage activity with manganese over magnesium. Noncoding RNA. 2020;**6**(1):14

[26] Symons RH. Plant pathogenic RNAs and RNA catalysis. Nucleic Acids Research. 1997;**25**(14):2683-2689

[27] Kuzmin YI, Da Costa CP, Fedor MJ. Role of an active site guanine in hairpin ribozyme catalysis probed by exogenous nucleobase rescue. Journal of Molecular Biology. 2004;**340**(2):233-251

[28] Moosbauer J, Tabler M. A helix 1-extended hairpin ribozyme exhibits altered cleavage behavior in vitro. Antisense & Nucleic Acid Drug Development. 1997;**7**(2):79-87

[29] Paudel BP, Rueda D. Molecular crowding accelerates ribozyme docking and catalysis. Journal of the American Chemical Society. 2014;**136**(48):16700-16703

[30] Netter HJ, Barrios MH, Littlejohn M, Yuen LKW. Hepatitis Delta Virus (HDV) and delta-like agents: Insights into their origin. Frontiers in Microbiology. 2021;**12**:652962

[31] Ferré-D, Amaré AR, Zhou K, Doudna JA. Crystal structure of a hepatitis delta virus ribozyme. Nature. 1998;**395**(6702):567-574

[32] Ferré-D, Amaré AR. The glmS ribozyme: Use of a small molecule co-enzyme by a gene-regulatory RNA. Quarterly Reviews of Biophysics. 2010;**43**(4):423-447

[33] Soukup J. The glmS ribozyme and its multifunctional coenzyme glucosamine-6-phosphate. Ribozymes. 2021;**2021**:91-115

[34] McCown PJ, Winkler WC, Breaker RR. Mechanism and distribution of glmS ribozymes. Methods in Molecular Biology. 2012;**848**:113-129

[35] Bingaman JL, Gonzalez IY, Wang B, Bevilacqua PC. Activation of the glmS ribozyme nucleophile via overdetermined hydrogen bonding. Biochemistry. 2017;**56**(33):4313-4317

[36] Suslov NB, DasGupta S, Huang H, Fuller JR, Lilley DM, Rice PA, et al. Crystal structure of the Varkud satellite ribozyme. Nature Chemical Biology. 2015;**11**(11):840-846

[37] Lafontaine DA, Norman DG, Lilley DM. Structure, folding and activity of the VS ribozyme: Importance of the 2-3-6 helical junction. The EMBO Journal. 2001;**20**(6):1415-1424

[38] Zheng L, Falschlunger C, Huang K, Mairhofer E, Yuan S, Wang J, et al. Hatchet ribozyme structure and implications for cleavage mechanism. Proceedings of the National Academy of Sciences. 2019;**116**(22):10783-10791

[39] Li S, Lünse CE, Harris KA, Breaker RR. Biochemical analysis of hatchet self-cleaving ribozymes. RNA. 2015;**21**(11):1845-1851

[40] Felletti M, Stifel J, Wurmthaler LA, Geiger S, Hartig JS. Twister ribozymes as highly versatile expression platforms for artificial riboswitches. Nature Communications. 2016;**7**(1):12834

[41] Wilson TJ, Liu Y, Domnick C, Kath-Schorr S, Lilley DMJ. The novel chemical mechanism of the twister ribozyme. Journal of the American Chemical Society. 2016;**138**(19):6151-6162

[42] Świderek K, Marti S, Tuñón I, Moliner V, Bertran J. Molecular mechanism of the site-specific self-cleavage of the RNA phosphodiester backbone by a twister ribozyme. Theoretical Chemistry Accounts. 2017;**136**(3):31

[43] Gasser C, Gebetsberger J, Gebetsberger M, Micura R. SHAPE probing pictures Mg2+-dependent folding of small self-cleaving ribozymes. Nucleic Acids Research. 2018;**46**(14):6983-6995

[44] Zheng L, Mairhofer E, Teplova M, Zhang Y, Ma J, Patel DJ, et al. Structure-based insights into self-cleavage by a four-way junctional twister-sister ribozyme. Nature Communications. 2017;**8**(1):1180

[45] Nguyen LA, Wang J, Steitz TA. Crystal structure of Pistol, a class of self-cleaving ribozyme. Proceedings of the National Academy of Sciences. 2017;**114**(5):1021-1026

[46] Harris KA, Lünse CE, Li S, Brewer KI, Breaker RR. Biochemical analysis of pistol self-cleaving ribozymes. RNA. 2015;**21**(11):1852-1858

[47] Peng H, Latifi B, Müller S, Lupták A, Chen IA. Self-cleaving ribozymes: Substrate specificity and synthetic biology applications. RSC Chemical Biology. 2021;**2**(5):1370-1383

[48] Chen Y, Qi F, Gao F, Cao H, Xu D, Salehi-Ashtiani K, et al. Hovlinc is a recently evolved class of ribozyme found in human lncRNA. Nature Chemical Biology. 2021;**17**(5):601-607

[49] Lykke-Andersen J, Aagaard C, Semionenkov M, Garrett RA. Archaeal introns: Splicing, intercellular mobility and evolution. Trends in Biochemical Sciences. 1997;**22**(9):326-331

[50] Cech TR. Self-splicing of group I introns. Annual Review of Biochemistry. 1990;**59**:543-568

[51] Lambowitz AM, Belfort M. Introns as mobile genetic elements. Annual Review of Biochemistry. 1993;**62**:587-622

[52] Michel F, Westhof E. Modelling of the three-dimensional architecture of group I catalytic introns based on comparative sequence analysis. Journal of Molecular Biology. 1990;**216**(3):585-610

[53] Matsuura M, Saldanha R, Ma H, Wank H, Yang J, Mohr G, et al.

A bacterial group II intron encoding reverse transcriptase, maturase, and DNA endonuclease activities: Biochemical demonstration of maturase activity and insertion of new genetic information within the intron. Genes & Development. 1997;**11**(21):2910-2924

[54] Pyle AM. Intron Self-Splicing. Annual Review of Biophysics. 2016;**45**:183-205

[55] Darr SC, Brown JW, Pace NR. The varieties of ribonuclease P. Trends in Biochemical Sciences. 1992;**17**(5):178-182

[56] Pace NR, Brown JW. Evolutionary perspective on the structure and function of ribonuclease P, a ribozyme. Journal of Bacteriology. 1995;**177**(8):1919-1928

[57] Persson T, Cuzic S, Hartmann RK. Catalysis by RNase P RNA: Unique features and unprecedented active site plasticity. The Journal of Biological Chemistry. 2003;**278**(44):43394-43401

[58] Klemm BP, Wu N, Chen Y, Liu X, Kaitany KJ, Howard MJ, et al. The Diversity of ribonuclease P: Protein and RNA catalysts with analogous biological functions. Biomolecules. 2016;**6**(2):27

[59] Will CL, Lührmann R. Spliceosome structure and function. Cold Springer Herbal Perspective Biology. 2011;**3**(7):a003707

[60] Wan R, Bai R, Zhan X, Shi Y. How is precursor messenger RNA spliced by the spliceosome? Annual Review of Biochemistry. 2020;**89**:333-358

[61] Wilkinson ME, Charenton C, Nagai K. RNA splicing by the spliceosome. Annual Review of Biochemistry. 2020;**89**:359-388

[62] Monachello D, Michel F, Costa M. Activating the branch-forming splicing pathway by reengineering the ribozyme component of a natural group II intron. RNA. 2016;**22**(3):443-455

[63] Wilson DN, Doudna Cate JH. The structure and function of the eukaryotic ribosome. Cold Springer Herbal Perspective Biology. 2012;**4**(5):a011536

[64] Alonso D, Mondragón A. Mechanisms of catalytic RNA molecules. Biochemical Society Transactions. 2021;**49**(4):1529-1535

[65] Tirumalai MR, Rivas M, Tran Q, Fox GE. The peptidyl transferase center: A window to the past. Microbiology and Molecular Biology Reviews. 2021;**85**(4):e0010421

[66] Kilani AF, Trang P, Jo S, Hsu A, Kim J, Nepomuceno E, et al. RNase P ribozymes selected in vitro to cleave a viral mRNA effectively inhibit its expression in cell culture. The Journal of Biological Chemistry. 2000;**275**(14):10611-10622

[67] Trang P, Lee J, Kilani AF, Kim J, Liu F. Effective inhibition of herpes simplex virus 1 gene expression and growth by engineered RNase P ribozyme. Nucleic Acids Research. 2001;**29**(24):5071-5078

[68] Watson ZL, Washington SD, Phelan DM, Lewin AS, Tuli SS, Schultz GS, et al. In vivo knockdown of the herpes simplex virus 1 latency-associated transcript reduces reactivation from latency. Journal of Virology. 2018;**92**(16):e00812-18

[69] Kim K, Umamoto S, Trang P, Hai R, Liu F. Intracellular expression of engineered RNase P ribozymes effectively blocks gene expression and replication of human cytomegalovirus. RNA. 2004;**10**(3):438-447

[70] Bai Y, Trang P, Li H, Kim K, Zhou T, Liu F. Effective inhibition in animals of viral pathogenesis by a ribozyme derived from RNase P catalytic RNA. Proceedings

of the National Academy of Sciences. 2008;**105**(31):10919-10924

[71] Bai Y, Gong H, Li H, Vu G-P, Lu S, Liu F. Oral delivery of RNase P ribozymes by *Salmonella* inhibits viral infection in mice. Proceedings of the National Academy of Sciences. 2011;**108**(8):3222-3227

[72] Sun X, Chen W, He L, Sheng J, Liu Y, Vu GP, et al. Inhibition of human cytomegalovirus immediate early gene expression and growth by a novel RNase P ribozyme variant. PLoS One. 2017;**12**(10):e0186791

[73] Li W, Liu Y, Wang Y, Li R, Trang P, Tang W, et al. Engineered RNase P ribozymes effectively inhibit the infection of murine cytomegalovirus in animals. Theranostics. 2018;**8**(20):5634-5644

[74] Amado RG, Mitsuyasu RT, Rosenblatt JD, Ngok FK, Bakker A, Cole S, et al. Anti-human immunodeficiency virus hematopoietic progenitor cell-delivered ribozyme in a phase I study: Myeloid and lymphoid reconstitution in human immunodeficiency virus type-1-infected patients. Human Gene Therapy. 2004;**15**(3):251-262

[75] Fedoruk-Wyszomirska A, Szymański M, Wyszko E, Barciszewska MZ, Barciszewski J. Highly active low magnesium hammerhead ribozyme. Journal of Biochemistry. 2009;**145**(4):451-459

[76] Zeng W, Chen Y-C, Bai Y, Trang P, Vu G-P, Lu S, et al. Effective inhibition of human immunodeficiency virus 1 replication by engineered RNase P Ribozyme. PLoS One. 2012;7(12):e51855

[77] Fedoruk-Wyszomirska A, Szymański M, Głodowicz P, Gabryelska M, Wyszko E, Estrin WJ, et al. Inhibition of HIV-1 gp41 expression with hammerhead ribozymes. The Biochemical Journal. 2015;**471**(1):53-66

[78] Motard J, Rouxel R, Paun A, von Messling V, Bisaillon M, Perreault J-P. A novel ribozyme-based prophylaxis inhibits Influenza A virus replication and protects from severe disease. PLoS One. 2011;**6**(11):e27327

[79] Czapik T, Piasecka J, Kierzek R, Kierzek E. Structural variants and modifications of hammerhead ribozymes targeting influenza A virus conserved structural motifs. Molecular Therapy--Nucleic Acids. 2022;**29**:64-74

[80] Seyhan AA, Vitiello D, Shields MT, Burke JM. Ribozyme inhibition of alphavirus replication. The Journal of Biological Chemistry. 2002;**277**(29):25957-25962

[81] Zhang Z, Burke JM. Inhibition of viral replication by ribozyme: Mutational analysis of the site and mechanism of antiviral activity. Journal of Virology. 2005;**79**(6):3728-3736

[82] Mishra P, Furey C, Balaraman V, Fraser MJ. Antiviral hammerhead ribozymes are effective for developing transgenic suppression of chikungunya virus in Aedes aegypti Mosquitoes. Viruses. 2016;**8**(6):163

[83] Mao X, Li X, Mao X, Huang Z, Zhang C, Zhang W, et al. Inhibition of hepatitis C virus by an M1GS ribozyme derived from the catalytic RNA subunit of Escherichia coli RNase P. Virology Journal. 2014;**11**:86

[84] Fukushima A, Fukuda N, Lai Y, Ueno T, Moriyama M, Taguchi F, et al. development of a chimeric DNA-RNA hammerhead ribozyme targeting SARS virus. Intervirology. 2009;**52**(2):92-99

[85] Felletti M, Bieber A, Hartig JS. The 3’-untranslated region of mRNAs as a site for ribozyme cleavage-dependent

processing and control in bacteria. RNA Biology. 2017;**14**(11):1522-1533

[86] Kogan M, Rappaport J. HIV-1 Accessory Protein Vpr: Relevance in the pathogenesis of HIV and potential for therapeutic intervention. Retrovirology. 2011;**8**(1):25

[87] Rice AP. The HIV-1 Tat protein: Mechanism of action and target for HIV-1 cure strategies. Current Pharmaceutical Design. 2017;**23**(28):4098-4102

[88] Macpherson JL, Boyd MP, Arndt AJ, Todd AV, Fanning GC, Ely JA, et al. Long-term survival and concomitant gene expression of ribozyme-transduced CD4+ T-lymphocytes in HIV-infected patients. The Journal of Gene Medicine. 2005;**7**(5):552-564

[89] Fernandes J, Jayaraman B, Frankel A. The HIV-1 Rev response element: An RNA scaffold that directs the cooperative assembly of a homo-oligomeric ribonucleoprotein complex. RNA Biology. 2012;**9**(1):6-11

[90] Pavco PA, Bouhana KS, Gallegos AM, Agrawal A, Blanchard KS, Grimm SL, et al. Antitumor and antimetastatic activity of ribozymes targeting the messenger RNA of vascular endothelial growth factor receptors. Clinical Cancer Research. 2000;**6**(5):2094-2103

[91] Weng DE, Masci PA, Radka SF, Jackson TE, Weiss PA, Ganapathi R, et al. A phase I clinical trial of a ribozyme-based angiogenesis inhibitor targeting vascular endothelial growth factor receptor-1 for patients with refractory solid tumors. Molecular Cancer Therapeutics. 2005;**4**(6):948-955

[92] Kobayashi H, Gail Eckhardt S, LockridgeJA,RothenbergML,SandlerAB,O, BryantCL,etal.Safetyandpharmacokinetic study of RPI.4610 (ANGIOZYME), an anti-VEGFR-1 ribozyme, in combination with carboplatin and paclitaxel in patients with advanced solid tumors. Cancer Chemotherapy and Pharmacology. 2005;**56**(4):329-336

[93] Morrow PK, Murthy RK, Ensor JD, Gordon GS, Margolin KA, Elias AD, et al. An open-label, phase 2 trial of RPI.4610 (angiozyme) in the treatment of metastatic breast cancer. Cancer. 2012;**118**(17):4098-4104

[94] Schmidt C, Welz R, Müller S. RNA double cleavage by a hairpin-derived twin ribozyme. Nucleic Acids Research. 2000;**28**(4):886-894

[95] Tijerina P, Mohr S, Russell R. DMS footprinting of structured RNAs and RNA-protein complexes. Nature Protocols. 2007;**2**(10):2608-2623

[96] Peattie DA, Gilbert W. Chemical probes for higher-order structure in RNA. Proceedings of the National Academy of Sciences. 1980;**77**(8):4679-4682

[97] Waduge P, Sakakibara Y, Chow CS. Chemical probing for examining the structure of modified RNAs and ligand binding to RNA. Methods. 2019;**156**:110-120

[98] Kharma N, Varin L, Abu-Baker A, Ouellet J, Najeh S, Ehdaeivand M-R, et al. Automated design of hammerhead ribozymes and validation by targeting the PABPN1 gene transcript. Nucleic Acids Research. 2016;**44**(4):e39

[99] Lucier J-F, Bergeron LJ, Brière FP, Ouellette R, Elela SA, Perreault J-P. RiboSubstrates: A web application addressing the cleavage specificities of ribozymes in designated genomes. BMC Bioinformatics. 2006;**7**(1):480

[100] Dotu I, Garcia-Martin JA, Slinger BL, Mechery V, Meyer MM, Clote P. Complete RNA inverse folding:

Computational design of functional hammerhead ribozymes. Nucleic Acids Research. 2014;**42**(18):11752-11762

[101] Chen X, Li N, Ellington AD. Ribozyme catalysis of metabolism in the RNA world. Chemistry & Biodiversity. 2007;**4**(4):633-655

[102] Barroso-DelJesus A, Berzal-Herranz A. Selection of targets and the most efficient hairpin ribozymes for inactivation of mRNAs using a self-cleaving RNA library. EMBO Reports. 2001;**2**(12):1112-1118

[103] Maghami MG, Scheitl CPM, Höbartner C. Direct in vitro selection of trans-acting ribozymes for posttranscriptional, site-specific, and covalent fluorescent labeling of RNA. Journal of the American Chemical Society. 2019;**141**(50):19546-19549

[104] Kobori S, Yokobayashi Y. Analyzing and tuning ribozyme activity by deep sequencing to modulate gene expression level in mammalian cells. ACS Synthetic Biology. 2018;**7**(2):371-376

[105] Yokobayashi Y. High-throughput analysis and engineering of ribozymes and deoxyribozymes by sequencing. Accounts of Chemical Research. 2020;**53**(12):2903-2912

[106] Samanta B, Joyce GF. A reverse transcriptase ribozyme. eLife. 2017;**6**:e31153

[107] Winkler WC, Nahvi A, Roth A, Collins JA, Breaker RR. Control of gene expression by a natural metabolite-responsive ribozyme. Nature. 2004;**428**(6980):281-286

[108] Denesyuk NA, Thirumalai D. How do metal ions direct ribozyme folding? Nature Chemistry. 2015;7(10):793-801

[109] Christiansen JK, Lobedanz S, Arar K, Wengel J, Vester B. LNA nucleotides improve cleavage efficiency of singular and binary hammerhead ribozymes. Bioorganic & Medicinal Chemistry. 2007;**15**(18):6135-6143

[110] Rouge JL, Sita TL, Hao L, Kouri FM, Briley WE, Stegh AH, et al. Ribozyme–spherical nucleic acids. Journal of the American Chemical Society. 2015;**137**(33):10528-10531

[111] Aigner A, Fischer D, Merdan T, Brus C, Kissel T, Czubayko F. Delivery of unmodified bioactive ribozymes by an RNA-stabilizing polyethylenimine (LMW-PEI) efficiently down-regulates gene expression. Gene Therapy. 2002;**9**(24):1700-1707

[112] Lau MWL, Ferré-D, Amaré AR. An in vitro evolved glmS ribozyme has the wild-type fold but loses co-enzyme dependence. Nature Chemical Biology. 2013;**9**(12):805-810

[113] Mitsuyasu RT, Merigan TC, Carr A, Zack JA, Winters MA, Workman C, et al. Phase 2 gene therapy trial of an anti-HIV ribozyme in autologous CD34+ cells. Nature Medicine. 2009;**15**(3):285-292

[114] Peng Y, Ai X, Peng B. Trans-cleaving hammerhead ribozyme in specific regions can improve knockdown efficiency in vivo. Journal of Cellular Biochemistry. 2022:1-10

[115] Borda EJ, Sigurdsson ST. Investigation of Mg2+- and temperature-dependent folding of the hairpin ribozyme by photo-crosslinking: Effects of photo-crosslinker tether length and chemistry. Nucleic Acids Research. 2005;**33**(3):1058-1068

[116] Burke DH, Greathouse ST. Low-magnesium, trans-cleavage activity by type III, tertiary stabilised hammerhead

ribozymes with stem 1 discontinuities. BMC Biochemistry. 2005;**6**(1):14

[117] Truong D et al. Enhanced group II intron retrohoming in magnesium-deficient Escherichia coli via selection of mutations in the ribozyme core. Proceedings of the National Academy of Sciences. 2013;**110**(40):E3800-E3900

Section 3

Anti-Cancer RNA Therapeutics

Chapter 4

A New Era of RNA Personalized Vaccines for Cancer and Cancer-Causing Infectious Diseases

Ana Ayala Pazzi, Puneet Vij, Nura Salhadar, Elias George and Manish K. Tripathi

Abstract

RNA vaccines for cancer and cancer-causing infectious agents are recognized as new therapeutics and are perceived as potential alternatives to conventional vaccines. Cancer is a leading cause of death worldwide, and infections (certain viruses, bacteria, and parasites) are linked to about 15–20% of cancers. Since the last decade, developments in genomics methodologies have provided a valuable tool to analyze the specific mutations, fusions, and translocations of the driver genes in specific cancer tissues. The landscape of the mutations identified by genome sequencing and data analysis can be a vital route to personalized medicine. This chapter will discuss the present state of mRNA vaccine development and ongoing clinical trials in oncology.

Keywords: mRNA, therapeutics, cancer, clinical trials, vaccine

1. Introduction

Conventional vaccine approaches were adopted for infectious diseases, but the RNA (mRNA) vaccine developed for COVID-19 changed the vaccine development landscape, providing global recognition and a new alternative. Moreover, RNA vaccines consist of rapid development, scalability, and cell-free manufacturing [1]. RNA vaccines are the clinical reality and are being studied to treat cancer, diseases like HIV, influenza, and genetic disorders [2]. mRNA cancer vaccines have received lots of attention, and efforts have resulted in some rapid developments, especially in the last 5 years [3, 4].

Cancer is not an infectious disease; vaccines for cancer aim to clear active disease instead of preventing disease, the only exception being the recently approved vaccine that prevents cancers caused by the human papillomavirus (HPV) [5]. Cancer is a particularly unpredictable disease that occurs due to random genetic events, and mutations are the driving force [6, 7]. Even though most potentially detrimental mutations are eliminated or neutral in nature, one mutation may cause a single somatic cell to develop an advantage over the rest, generating a pattern of amplified proliferation and progression that, over time, gives rise to a cancerous tumor [8]. Genome profiling provides insight into the diversity and heterogeneity within each type of cancer, which is a significant challenge in finding the right therapy for each patient [9, 10].

1.1 What is mRNA?

Messenger RNA is a versatile, single-stranded molecule that mediates protein translation, posttranscriptionally regulates genes, and has other regulatory properties inside the cell [11, 12]. A mature mRNA will have a protein-encoding region, or open reading frame (ORF), between a start and a stop codon enclosed in a single strand with a 7-methyl-guanosine and untranslated region at the 5′ end and a poly-A tail with its respective untranslated region at the 3′ end. Both the 5′ cap and the poly-A tail are essential for mRNA maturation and stability, therefore heavily regulating the efficiency of protein translation and mRNA degradation [13, 14]. Generally, once the mRNA enters the cell, it has a short time to produce the protein it is encoding for before it starts to degrade [15]. This is a challenge when studying mRNA as a therapeutic delivery, especially in hereditary diseases [16, 17].

1.2 RNA therapeutics

mRNA presents a viable option for patient therapeutics comparable to existing cancer therapies [13, 18]. Since the inception of RNA-based cancer vaccination, many preclinical and clinical studies have explored the idea of mRNA-based anticancer vaccines using autologous RNA-transfected dendritic cells or direct injection into the organism. For instance, mRNA acts outside the cell nucleus, eliminating the need to bypass this membrane while still being a messenger for genetic information. In the cytoplasm, the exogenously delivered mRNA starts protein translation, whereas DNA must reach the nucleus first and then be transcribed into mRNA to produce an effect in the cell [15 19, 20]. Additionally, mRNA does not incorporate into the genome; instead, it produces proteins for a short period, significantly minimizing the risk of mutations in the patient and long-term side effects [21]. Moreover, mRNA drugs can be manufactured relatively inexpensively to express any protein for virtually any disease. Multiple research studies conducted during the past few decades have demonstrated the curative properties of this technology and its ability to target various health conditions [22–25]. This is particularlytrue in the case of synthetic mRNA-based vaccines that were developed rapidly

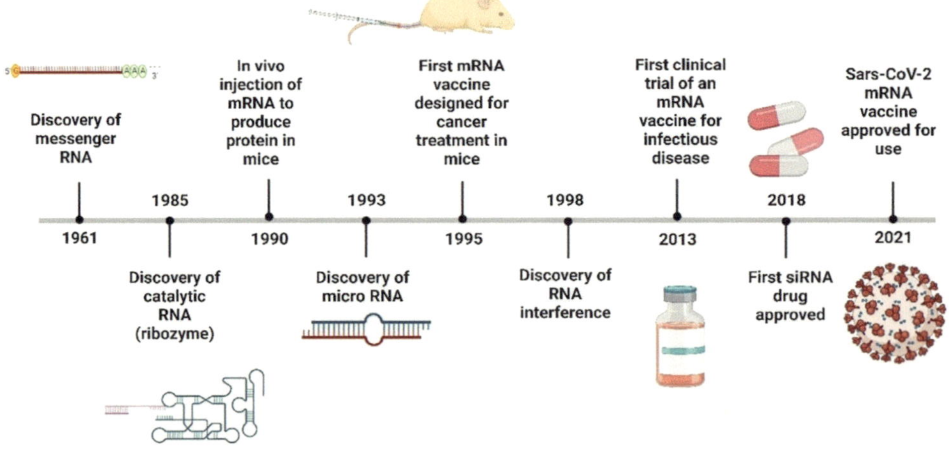

Figure 1.
Key discoveries and advances in mRNA-based therapeutics. Created with BioRender.com.

during the COVID-19 pandemic, and many years of research in RNA biology paved the way for this unparalleled achievement. The first mRNA vaccine approved for emergency use for infectious disease (COVID-19) by the FDA was created by BioNTech and Pfizer [26]. The candidates for the vaccine (BNT162b1 and BNT162B2) were initially identified in Germany and were further studied in the United States [27]. These targets were chosen as they encoded the spike protein of the SARS-CoV-2 virus. The delivery method for this vaccine consisted of lipid nanoparticles [28]. The Moderna vaccine also targeted a similar gene product and was delivered intramuscularly to the patient. **Figure 1** shows the history of RNA and the recent development of mRNA-based COVID-19 vaccines.

2. Challenges and advantages of mRNA vaccines

The delivery of mRNA into a cell is particularly challenging due to the size of 300 to 5000 bp, in contrast to microRNA and silencing RNA, which only go up to 5–15 bp in size. Additionally, instability due to charges in the molecule is another factor that impairs its functionality as a therapy, as it cannot penetrate the cell membrane. However, some cells can uptake naked mRNA, a relatively inefficient process, because most cells have a low rate of mRNA uptake [29, 30]. In contrast, the immature dendritic cell is an exception, which can take up mRNA through the macro pinocytosis pathway and accumulate mRNA efficiently [15].

One advantage of mRNA vaccines is a simplified development process, which only requires a few laboratory techniques and resources. In contrast, the production of biologics such as plasmid DNA vaccines can be time-consuming and expensive compared to mRNA vaccines, thereby augmenting the interest in mRNA therapeutics. However, in the initial stages of the study surrounding mRNA vaccines, researchers struggled to stabilize the product and increase its safety profile [31, 32]. Some solutions to these issues included chemical modification of mRNA sequences (e.g., via nucleoside manipulations) and packaging into nanocarriers [33, 34]. RNA-active vaccines (protamine-formulated mRNA vaccines) encoding six prostate cancer-specific antigens (CV9104) and five non-small cell lung cancer (NSCLC) tumor-associated antigens (CV9201) have been investigated clinically for safety, overall survival, and progression-free survival [35].

The challenges that must be overcome in the production of mRNA vaccines include the negative charge of the RNA (which must cross the hydrophobic cell membrane) and the strong immune reaction of exogenous RNA, which can cause cell toxicity [29, 36]. Recent research has overcome these obstacles by personalization of vaccines for their ability to target specific diseases [16, 37]. Moreover, once synthetic mRNA is translated into protein in the cytoplasm, it is subsequently degraded within a few minutes or hours, thereby preventing any harmful effects.

Various forms of mRNA therapy include replacement therapy (to synthesize a defective protein), vaccination, and cell therapy (which entails ex vivo transfection) [16]. Another challenge is that antigen presentation is often short-lived, as mRNA can be degraded by exogenous RNases [21]. However, this can be addressed using self-amplifying RNA sequences utilized by alphaviruses, which prolong antigen expression [38].

3. Immunology of vaccination

The human immune system is comprised of innate and adaptive immune cells that play unique roles in eliminating a pathogen. The innate immune system serves as a first-line response to a pathogen and acts via lysis or phagocytosis [39, 40]. Since it is possible for pathogens to evade this first-line defense, the adaptive immune system can prompt the activation of humoral and cell-mediated immunity (see **Table 1**) [33, 41]. Humoral immunity consists of B-cells that produce antibodies, which can eliminate a pathogen via various mechanisms. Antibodies may envelop the pathogen with their Fc (constant fragment) portions which are subsequently recognized by phagocytic cells [42]. Other mechanisms include the creation of immune complexes which trigger the complement cascade, expressing receptors on phagocytic cells and directly attaching antibodies to viruses via receptor binding sites [33]. Cell-mediated

Immune response	Immune product	Infectious agents
Humoral	Immunoglobulin G	Bacteria and viruses
	Immunoglobulin A	Microorganisms
	Immunoglobulin M	Bacteria
	Immunoglobulin E	Parasites
Cell-mediated	Cytotoxic T-lymphocyte	Viruses, mycobacteria, parasites
	T-helper cells 1	Mycobacteria, fungi

Table 1.
Immune response, products, and associated infectious diseases [33].

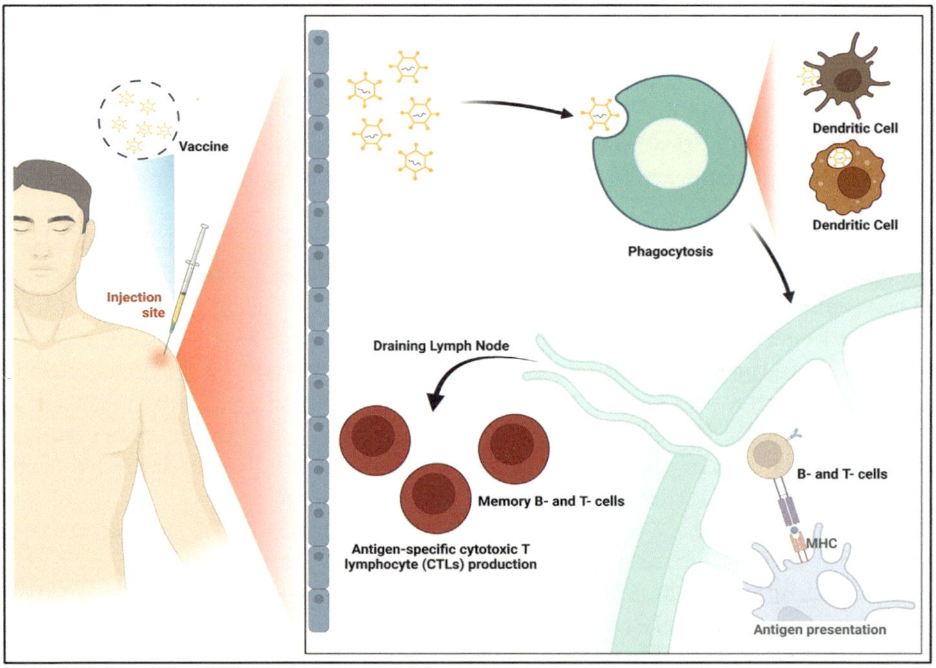

Figure 2.
Administration of vaccine leading to immunity production steps. Macrophages and dendritic cells are phagocytic antigen-presenting cells (APCs). Upon vaccine administration, these APCs take up the contents of the vaccine. After activation of APCs by specific antigens, the migration occurs toward lymph nodes (LNs) as shown. Within the LNs, the antigen is presented to lymphocytes for further activation. Antigen-specific B- and T-cells then multiply clonally to create their progenitors by recognizing the same antigen. Long-term protection is also achieved by the production of memory B- and T-cells against pathogen infection. Created with BioRender.com.

immunity clears infected cells via cytotoxic T-cells and T-helper cells. The B- and T-cells of the adaptive immune system are more specific to the pathogen, and vaccines seek to build up this response to evade the severe consequences of infection. Upon infection, the innate immune system prompts B-cells and T-cells (specific to the virus) increase in number, thereby strengthening their degree of protection [33, 43]. The vaccine entry requires uptake *via* antigen-presenting cells, which deliver the vaccine to secondary lymphoid organs where T- and B-cells are produced (see **Figure 2**).

Once the infection has cleared, some of the B- and T-cells will undergo apoptosis, but some may persist and will be able to respond if re-infection of the same pathogen

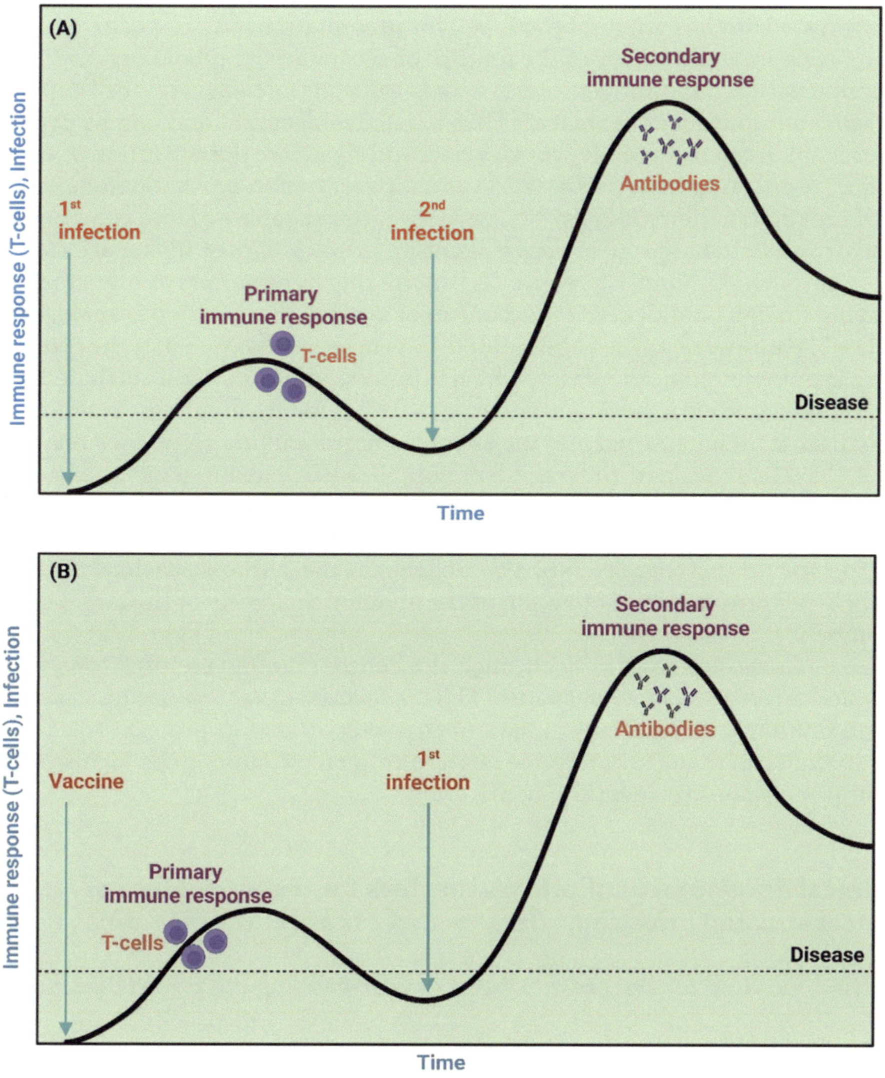

Figure 3.
Adaptive immune responses after two different scenarios: (A) infection: This part of the figure represents the response after primary and secondary infection. The primary infection causes disease manifestation, as there is a lag in developing T- and B-cells. The secondary infection causes the memory T-cells to respond quickly and helps develop antibodies to fight the infection or pathogen. (B) Administration of vaccination follows a similar pattern without the manifestation of the disease. Created with BioRender.com.

occurs (see **Figure 3**). Thus, the aim of achieving a faster immunological response to a pathogen is achieved through this mechanism [44].

For effective antibody production, the coordinated actions of CD4-positive follicular helper T-cells and B-cells depend on the successful presentation of a protein antigen, which is recognized by its specific B-cell clone in secondary lymphoid organs such as the lymph node and provides the first signal for B-cell activation [45]. This specific B-cell clone processes an extracellular protein antigen by uptake into endosomes and lysosomes for proteolytic digestion into peptides of varying length for incorporation into highly diverse HLA Class II molecules, which are imported from the endoplasmic reticulum [46] and can bind antigenic peptides of 10 to 30 residues in length. The mature HLA Class II molecule bearing its antigenic peptide is then expressed on the surface of the B-cell for presentation to CD4-positive follicular helper T-cells at the periphery of the follicles of secondary lymphoid organs. The interaction between the antigen-presenting B-cell and the follicular T-cell depends on specific recognition of the mature HLA Class II molecule containing its peptide antigen by its T-cell receptor. It provides a second signal for the activation of the B lymphocyte resulting in its proliferation and differentiation into antibody-secreting plasma cells and memory B-cells [47], with the latter capable of rapid response to a second exposure to its specific antigen resulting in antibodies of higher affinity.

Cell-mediated immunity targets cells functioning as reservoirs of infection or displaying foreign peptides. The mechanism of antigen presentation is analogous to the Class II pathway described above but differs in several ways. First, the protein antigen is present in the cytoplasm, which is processed by ubiquitin-mediated proteasomal digestion resulting in small peptide fragments about nine residues in length that are then imported into the endoplasmic reticulum. Here, they may bind to HLA Class I molecules if the fragments contain sufficient antigenicity. The mature HLA Class I molecules with their bound antigenic peptides are then displayed on the antigen-presenting cell surface for recognition by an activated CD8-positive cytotoxic T cell specific for this complex [48, 49]. Delivery of the cytotoxic payload of this effector T-cell results in the activation of the apoptotic pathway of the target cell and its elimination.

A second exposure to an antigen, such as a booster, is often required for a more robust and effective immune response. Thus, a successful vaccine design strategy requires this immunologic knowledge and characteristics of its protein target, where computational methods to determine peptide antigenicity among the highly polymorphic HLA molecules are helpful [50, 51].

4. Clinical development of mRNA vaccines for the prevention of cancer-causing infectious diseases and as cancer therapeutics

4.1 mRNA vaccines for the prevention of cancer-causing infectious diseases

Microbial infection accounts for around 15% of all human cancers, totaling approximately two million yearly cases [52]. Bacterium Helicobacter pylori, human papillomavirus (HPV), hepatitis B virus (HBV), hepatitis C virus (HCV), and Epstein–Barr virus (EBV) are primarily responsible for 97% of these cancers [53]. Besides cancer-causing infectious diseases, mRNA vaccines are also being studied as a preventive treatment against influenza A, zika, cytomegalovirus, respiratory syncytial, and rabies [16].

Currently, mRNA vaccines have been designed for two of seven viruses that can cause cancer (oncoviruses). One of the examples is the liposome-encapsulated mRNA vaccine for human papillomavirus type 16 (HPV-16). It encodes for the oncoproteins E6 and E7, which have the potential for immunomodulation and antineoplastic activities [54]. Upon intravenous administration, the liposomes protect the RNA degradation within the bloodstream leading to uptake by APCs [55]. Translocation to the cytoplasm leads to the translation of E6 and E7 oncoproteins. After the processing of the proteins, the peptide complexes are presented to the immune system and hence induce antigen-specific T-cell responses (CD8+ and CD4+) against HPV16 E6 and E7 [56]. The associated clinical trial is mentioned in **Table 2**. Another example is mRNA-1189 Epstein–Barr virus (EBV) vaccine. This encodes EBV's envelope glycoproteins (gH, gL, gp42, and gp220), which mediate viral entry into B-cells and epithelial surface cells, the primary targets of EBV infection [57, 58]. The viral proteins in mRNA-1189 are expressed in their native membrane-bound form for recognition by the human immune system.

Brand	Title	Conditions	Phase
BNT111	Trial with BNT111 and Cemiplimab as a single agent and/or in combination	Melanoma stage III/ and/or IV	Phase II
BNT112	Prostate Cancer Messenger RNA Immunotherapy	Prostate cancer	Phase I and II
BNT113	Safety, tolerability, and therapeutic effects of bnt113 in combination with Pembrolizumab/ Alone for participants with head/neck cancer positive for HPV16 and PD-L1 expression	Head and neck cancer	Phase II
BNT116	Clinical trial evaluating the safety, tolerability, and preliminary efficacy of BNT116 alone and/ or in combination	Non-small cell lung cancer	Phase I
BNT122	Comparing the efficacy of RO7198457 Vs. Watchful waiting in patients with high-risk stage II and Stage III colorectal cancer	Colorectal cancer Stage II/III	Phase II
RO7198457	A study of RO7198457 as a single agent and/or in combination with atezolizumab in participants with advanced or metastatic tumors	Melanoma Bladder cancer	Phase I
RO7198457	A study of the efficacy and safety of RO7198457 in combination with atezolizumab Vs. Atezolizumab alone	Non-small cell lung cancer	Phase II
RO7198457	A study to evaluate the efficacy and safety of RO7198457 in combination with pembrolizumab Vs. pembrolizumab alone in participants with previously untreated advanced melanoma	Advanced melanoma	Phase II
mRNA-4157	Safety, tolerability, and immunogenicity of mRNA-4157 alone in participants with resected solid tumors and/or in combination with pembrolizumab in participants with unresectable solid tumors	Solid tumors	Phase I
	An efficacy study of adjuvant treatment with the personalized cancer vaccine mRNA-4157 and pembrolizumab in participants with high-risk Melanoma	Melanoma	Phase II

Brand	Title	Conditions	Phase
mRNA5671/ V941	A study of mRNA-5671/V941 as monotherapy and in combination with pembrolizumab	Non-small cell lung cancer Pancreatic and colorectal Neoplasms	Phase I
mRNA-2752	Dose escalation study of mRNA-2752 for intra-tumoral injection to participants with advanced malignancies	Relapsed/ refractory solid Tumor malignancies or lymphoma	Phase I
SW1115C3	A study of neoantigen mRNA personalized cancer in patients with advanced solid tumors	Solid tumor	Phase I
mRNA-4539	Study of mRNA-4359 administered alone and in combination with Immune Checkpoint Blockade in participants with Advanced Solids Tumors	Advanced solid tumors	Phase I and II
BNT 141	Safety, pharmacokinetics, pharmacodynamics, and preliminary efficacy trial of BNT141 in patients with unresectable CLDN18.2-positive gastric, pancreatic, ovarian, and Biliary tract tumors	Solid tumor Gastric, pancreatic, biliary tract, and metastatic cancer	Phase I and IIa

Table 2.
Clinical trials of mRNA encoding TAAs and TSAs (clinical trials.gov).

Kaposi's sarcoma-associated herpesvirus (KSHV) is the cause of three human malignancies: Kaposi's sarcoma, primary effusion lymphoma, and the plasma cell variant of multicentric Castleman disease. Currently, there are no well-developed KSHV vaccine candidates. One of the clinical trials completed in 2019 looked at the impact of Valganciclovir on severe immune reconstitution syndrome (S-IRIS)-Kaposi Sarcoma (KS) mortality: an open-label, parallel, randomized controlled trial, in which 40 patients were randomized and 37 completed the study. It was concluded that Valganciclovir significantly reduced the episodes of S-IRIS-KS. Although attributable KS mortality was lower in the experimental group, the difference was insignificant. Mortality was significantly lower in EG patients with pulmonary KS [59].

4.2 Development of mRNA vaccines as cancer therapeutics

Several widely used conventional cancer therapies, such as chemotherapy and hormone therapy, have proven effective in treating cancer [60]. Chemotherapy involves a series of drugs that impair DNA synthesis, thus fatally interrupting the physiological processes of cancerous and healthy cells [61, 62]. However, the success rates for this treatment are most effective only in highly proliferative and low heterogeneity cancers. Alternatively, hormonal or endocrine therapy targets growth signaling pathways by interfering with hormone receptors in cancer cells [63]. Thus, it is suitable for low-proliferating cancers such as breast and prostate [64].

Among immunotherapeutic treatments, mRNA vaccines stand out due to their superior specificity and potential for adaptability according to the genetic profile of each patient's cancer. To produce an efficient, individualized cancer vaccine, specific genetic mutations in the cancerous cells are identified to produce neoantigens that could bind to T-cells and elicit an immune response in the patient more specifically than traditional systemic and local methods [37]. However, this treatment has faced challenges, such as a need to enhance the identification of potential genetic markers that could provide the specificity needed for cancer vaccines [23, 65].

RNA vaccines targeting various cancers are in the development and undergoing clinical trials. Examples of RNA cancer vaccines include CV9202 (CureVac), which targets multiple antigens found in non-small cell lung cancer [13]. Moderna is also developing an mRNA vaccine that targets the K-RAS proto-oncogene that plays a role in the pathogenesis of non-small cell lung cancer, colorectal cancer, and pancreatic adenocarcinoma [66]. The mRNA-4157 against melanoma, created by Moderna, and the BNT122 vaccine against prostate cancer, created by BioNTech, targets various solid tumors and are individualized vaccines [35, 67]. These specific vaccines are designed to elicit the immune response toward tumor-associated antigens (TAAs) or tumor-specific antigens (TSAs) in malignant tumor cells. These vaccines used next-generation sequencing technology to identify and isolate antigen epitopes unique to each patient, creating a more refined vaccine. Various clinical trials exist for different cancer vaccines (see **Table 2**) [2]. TAAs are present in both normal tissues and tumors, as these are non-mutated self-antigens. For a few tumors, TAAs are desirable vaccine targets. However, immune tolerance responses, such as central and peripheral, may be triggered by vaccines that can express TAAs and can reduce clinical vaccination efficacy [68]. Therefore, these kinds of vaccines are still in a phase where they are used in combination with immune checkpoint inhibitors [69]. With many ongoing clinical trials in different phases and preexisting clinical information or data, personalized vaccines can potentially be effective in cancer treatment. BioNTech vaccine BNT122 RO7198457) and Moderna vaccine mRNA-4157 are two personalized mRNA-based cancer vaccines in phase II clinical trials.

There is a significant increase in ongoing or completed studies/clinical trials in mRNA vaccines. In addition, various other clinical trials evaluate the tolerability, safety, immunogenicity, and/or efficacy of mRNA-personalized vaccines in participants with tumors. In this way, we are stepping into a new era of therapeutic mRNA-based cancer vaccines or prevention and treatment of currently incurable malignant diseases.

5. Summary

This chapter describes the technology, the basics of the immune response, and examples of developing mRNA vaccines for cancer and cancer-causing infectious agents. They can be used for preventive and therapeutic purposes. This information is of value to interdisciplinary researchers, engineers, and healthcare professionals as it may impact the prospects of medical care. Built on the highly fueled interest and potential, we have complete confidence to predict an accelerated pace in mRNA therapy studies and development in the next decade, possibly providing many solutions for the prevention and treatment of currently incurable diseases.

Funding acknowledgment

This study is supported by NIH/NIGMS R16GM146696 and UTRGV SOM Startup funds to MKT and partially supported by AARG-NTF Alzheimer's Association and KSA International Collaboration grant from Saudi Arabia to MKT.

Conflict of interest

The authors declare no conflict of interest.

Author details

Ana Ayala Pazzi[1,2†], Puneet Vij[3,4†], Nura Salhadar[5], Elias George[2,6] and Manish K. Tripathi[2,7*]

1 Department of Biology, College of Sciences, The University of Texas Rio Grande Valley, McAllen, TX, USA

2 Department of Immunology and Microbiology, School of Medicine, The University of Texas Rio Grande Valley, McAllen, TX, USA

3 Department of Pharmaceutical Sciences, St. John's University, Queens, NY, USA

4 Michigan Public Health Institute, Okemos, MI, USA

5 School of Medicine, The University of Texas Rio Grande Valley, Edinburgh, TX, USA

6 Department of Medical Education, School of Medicine, The University of Texas Rio Grande Valley, McAllen, TX, USA

7 South Texas Center of Excellence in Cancer Research, School of Medicine, The University of Texas Rio Grande Valley, McAllen, TX, USA

*Address all correspondence to: manish.tripathi@utrgv.edu

† Equal contribution.

References

[1] Bloom K, van den Berg F, Arbuthnot P. Self-amplifying RNA vaccines for infectious diseases. Gene Therapy. 2021;**28**(3-4):117-129. Epub 2020/10/24. DOI: 10.1038/s41434-020-00204-y

[2] Rosa SS, Prazeres DMF, Azevedo AM, Marques MPC. mRNA vaccines manufacturing: Challenges and bottlenecks. Vaccine. 2021;**39**(16):2190-2200. Epub 2021/03/28. DOI: 10.1016/j.vaccine.2021.03.038

[3] He Q, Gao H, Tan D, Zhang H, Wang JZ. mRNA cancer vaccines: Advances, trends and challenges. Acta Pharmaceutica Sinica B. 2022;**12**(7):2969-2989. Epub 2022/03/30. DOI: 10.1016/j.apsb.2022.03.011

[4] Chaudhary N, Weissman D, Whitehead KA. mRNA vaccines for infectious diseases: Principles, delivery and clinical translation. Nature Reviews Drug Discovery. 2021;**20**(11):817-838. Epub 2021/08/27. DOI: 10.1038/s41573-021-00283-5 K.A.W. is bound by confidential agreements that prevent her from disclosing related consulting relationships

[5] Paston SJ, Brentville VA, Symonds P, Durrant LG. Cancer vaccines, adjuvants, and delivery systems. Frontiers in Immunology. 2021;**12**:627932. Epub 2021/04/17. DOI: 10.3389/fimmu.2021.627932

[6] Feinberg AP. Epigenetic stochasticity, nuclear structure and cancer: The implications for medicine. Journal of Internal Medicine. 2014;**276**(1):5-11. Epub 2014/03/19. DOI: 10.1111/joim.12224

[7] Heng HH. Cancer genome sequencing: The challenges ahead. BioEssays: News and Reviews in Molecular, Cellular and Developmental Biology. 2007;**29**(8):783-794. Epub 2007/07/11. DOI: 10.1002/bies.20610

[8] Aktipis CA, Nesse RM. Evolutionary foundations for cancer biology. Evolutionary Applications. 2013;**6**(1):144-159. Epub 2013/02/12. DOI: 10.1111/eva.12034

[9] Turajlic S, Sottoriva A, Graham T, Swanton C. Author correction: Resolving genetic heterogeneity in cancer. Nature Reviews Genetics. 2020;**21**(1):65. Epub 2019/10/30. DOI: 10.1038/s41576-019-0188-1

[10] Dagogo-Jack I, Shaw AT. Tumour heterogeneity and resistance to cancer therapies. Nature Reviews Clinical oncology. 2018;**15**(2):81-94. Epub 2017/11/09. DOI: 10.1038/nrclinonc.2017.166

[11] Sanford JR, Gray NK, Beckmann K, Cáceres JF. A novel role for shuttling SR proteins in mRNA translation. Genes & Development. 2004;**18**(7):755-768. Epub 2004/04/15. DOI: 10.1101/gad.286404

[12] Kishore S, Luber S, Zavolan M. Deciphering the role of RNA-binding proteins in the post-transcriptional control of gene expression. Briefings in Functional Genomics. 2010;**9**(5-6):391-404. Epub 2010/12/04. DOI: 10.1093/bfgp/elq028

[13] Miao L, Zhang Y, Huang L. mRNA vaccine for cancer immunotherapy. Molecular Cancer. 2021;**20**(1):41. Epub 2021/02/27. DOI: 10.1186/s12943-021-01335-5

[14] Schlake T, Thess A, Fotin-Mleczek M, Kallen KJ. Developing mRNA-vaccine

technologies. RNA biology. 2012;**9**(11):1319-1330. Epub 2012/10/16. DOI: 10.4161/rna.22269

[15] Sahin U, Karikó K, Türeci Ö. mRNA-based therapeutics--developing a new class of drugs. Nature Reviews Drug discovery. 2014;**13**(10):759-780. Epub 2014/09/23. DOI: 10.1038/nrd4278

[16] Damase TR, Sukhovershin R, Boada C, Taraballi F, Pettigrew RI, Cooke JP. The limitless future of RNA therapeutics. Frontiers in Bioengineering and Biotechnology. 2021;**9**:628137. Epub 2021/04/06. DOI: 10.3389/fbioe.2021.628137

[17] Aagaard L, Rossi JJ. RNAi therapeutics: Principles, prospects and challenges. Advanced Drug Delivery Reviews. 2007;**59**(2-3):75-86. Epub 2007/04/24. DOI: 10.1016/j.addr.2007.03.005

[18] Wilson PM, Danenberg PV, Johnston PG, Lenz HJ, Ladner RD. Standing the test of time: Targeting thymidylate biosynthesis in cancer therapy. Nature Reviews Clinical Oncology. 2014;**11**(5):282-298. Epub 2014/04/16. DOI: 10.1038/nrclinonc.2014.51

[19] Schlake T, Thess A, Thran M, Jordan I. mRNA as novel technology for passive immunotherapy. Cellular and Molecular Life Sciences: CMLS. 2019;**76**(2):301-328. Epub 2018/10/20. DOI: 10.1007/s00018-018-2935-4

[20] Tomita T, Kato M, Mishima T, Matsunaga Y, Sanjo H, Ito KI, et al. Extracellular mRNA transported to the nucleus exerts translation-independent function. Nature Communications. 2021;**12**(1):3655. Epub 2021/06/18. DOI: 10.1038/s41467-021-23969-1

[21] Park JW, Lagniton PNP, Liu Y, Xu RH. mRNA vaccines for COVID-19: What, why and how. International Journal of Biological Sciences. 2021;**17**(6):1446-1460. Epub 2021/04/29. DOI: 10.7150/ijbs.59233

[22] Kim YK. RNA therapy: Rich history, various applications and unlimited future prospects. Experimental & Molecular Medicine. 2022;**54**(4):455-465. Epub 2022/04/21. DOI: 10.1038/s12276-022-00757-5

[23] Pardi N, Hogan MJ, Porter FW, Weissman D. mRNA vaccines - a new era in vaccinology. Nature Reviews Drug discovery. 2018;**17**(4):261-279. Epub 2018/01/13. DOI: 10.1038/nrd.2017.243

[24] Zhang C, Maruggi G, Shan H, Li J. Advances in mRNA vaccines for infectious diseases. Frontiers in Immunology. 2019;**10**:594. Epub 2019/04/12. DOI: 10.3389/fimmu.2019.00594

[25] Maruggi G, Zhang C, Li J, Ulmer JB, Yu D. mRNA as a transformative Technology for Vaccine Development to control infectious diseases. Molecular Therapy. 2019;**27**(4):757-772. Epub 2019/02/26. DOI: 10.1016/j.ymthe.2019.01.020

[26] Lamb YN. BNT162b2 mRNA COVID-19 vaccine: First approval. Drugs. 2021;**81**(4):495-501. Epub 2021/03/09. DOI: 10.1007/s40265-021-01480-7

[27] Khehra N, Padda I, Jaferi U, Atwal H, Narain S, Parmar MS. Tozinameran (BNT162b2) vaccine: The journey from preclinical research to clinical trials and authorization. AAPS Pharm Sci Tech. 2021;**22**(5):172. Epub 2021/06/09. DOI: 10.1208/s12249-021-02058-y

[28] Wilson B, Geetha KM. Lipid nanoparticles in the development of mRNA vaccines for COVID-19. Journal of Drug Delivery Science and Technology.

2022;**74**:103553. Epub 2022/07/06. DOI: 10.1016/j.jddst.2022.103553

[29] Zogg H, Singh R, Ro S. Current advances in RNA therapeutics for human diseases. International Journal of Molecular Sciences. 2022;**23**(5):2736. Epub 2022/03/11. DOI: 10.3390/ijms23052736

[30] Qin M, Du G, Sun X. Recent advances in the noninvasive delivery of mRNA. Accounts of Chemical Research. 2021;**54**(23):4262-4271. Epub 2021/11/11. DOI: 10.1021/acs.accounts.1c00493

[31] Jain S, Venkataraman A, Wechsler ME, Peppas NA. Messenger RNA-based vaccines: Past, present, and future directions in the context of the COVID-19 pandemic. Advanced Drug Delivery Reviews. 2021;**179**:114000. Epub 2021/10/13. DOI: 10.1016/j.addr.2021.114000

[32] Karim ME, Haque ST, Al-Busaidi H, Bakhtiar A, Tha KK, Holl MMB, et al. Scope and challenges of nanoparticle-based mRNA delivery in cancer treatment. Archives of Pharmacal Research. 2022;**45**(12):865-893. Epub 2022/11/25. DOI: 10.1007/s12272-022-01418-x

[33] Jiskoot WKG, Mastrobattista E, Slütter B. Vaccines. In: Pharmaceutical Biotechnology. Cham: Springer; 2019. pp. 281-304. DOI: 10.1007/978-3-030-00710-2_14

[34] Bost JP, Barriga H, Holme MN, Gallud A, Maugeri M, Gupta D, et al. Delivery of oligonucleotide therapeutics: Chemical modifications, lipid nanoparticles, and extracellular vesicles. ACS Nano. 2021;**15**(9):13993-14021. Epub 2021/09/11. DOI: 10.1021/acsnano.1c05099

[35] Lorentzen CL, Haanen JB, Met Ö, Svane IM. Clinical advances and ongoing trials on mRNA vaccines for cancer treatment. The Lancet Oncology. 2022;**23**(10):e450-e4e8. Epub 2022/09/30. DOI: 10.1016/s1470-2045(22)00372-2

[36] Qin L, Zhang H, Zhou Y, Umeshappa CS, Gao H. Nanovaccine-based strategies to overcome challenges in the whole vaccination Cascade for tumor immunotherapy. Small (Weinheim an der Bergstrasse, Germany). 2021;**17**(28):e2006000. Epub 2021/03/27. DOI: 10.1002/smll.202006000

[37] Zhang Z, Lu M, Qin Y, Gao W, Tao L, Su W, et al. Neoantigen: A new breakthrough in tumor immunotherapy. Frontiers in Immunology. 2021;**12**:672356. Epub 2021/05/04. DOI: 10.3389/fimmu.2021.672356

[38] Lundstrom K. Self-amplifying RNA viruses as RNA vaccines. International Journal of Molecular Sciences. 2020;**21**(14):5130. Epub 2020/07/24. DOI: 10.3390/ijms21145130

[39] Marshall JS, Warrington R, Watson W, Kim HL. An introduction to immunology and immunopathology. Allergy, asthma, and clinical immunology. 2018;**14**(Suppl. 2):49. Epub 2018/09/29. DOI: 10.1186/s13223-018-0278-1

[40] Riera Romo M, Pérez-Martínez D, Castillo FC. Innate immunity in vertebrates: An overview. Immunology. 2016;**148**(2):125-139. Epub 2016/02/16. DOI: 10.1111/imm.12597

[41] Cooper N, Arnold DM. The effect of rituximab on humoral and cell mediated immunity and infection in the treatment of autoimmune diseases. British Journal of haematology. 2010;**149**(1):3-13. Epub 2010/02/16. DOI: 10.1111/j.1365-2141.2010.08076.x

[42] Taylor A, Foo SS, Bruzzone R, Dinh LV, King NJ, Mahalingam S. Fc receptors in antibody-dependent enhancement of viral infections. Immunological Reviews. 2015;**268**(1): 340-364. Epub 2015/10/27. DOI: 10.1111/imr.12367

[43] Iwasaki A, Pillai PS. Innate immunity to influenza virus infection. Nature reviews Immunology. 2014;**14**(5):315-328. Epub 2014/04/26. DOI: 10.1038/nri3665

[44] Welsh RM, Che JW, Brehm MA, Selin LK. Heterologous immunity between viruses. Immunological Reviews. 2010;**235**(1):244-266. Epub 2010/06/12. DOI: 10.1111/j.0105-2896.2010.00897.x

[45] Förster R, Schubel A, Breitfeld D, Kremmer E, Renner-Müller I, Wolf E, et al. CCR7 coordinates the primary immune response by establishing functional microenvironments in secondary lymphoid organs. Cell. 1999;**99**(1):23-33. Epub 1999/10/16. DOI: 10.1016/s0092-8674(00)80059-8

[46] Roche PA, Furuta K. The ins and outs of MHC class II-mediated antigen processing and presentation. Nature Reviews Immunology. 2015;**15**(4):203-216. Epub 2015/02/28. DOI: 10.1038/nri3818

[47] Ueno H, Banchereau J, Vinuesa CG. Pathophysiology of T follicular helper cells in humans and mice. Nature Immunology. 2015;**16**(2):142-152. Epub 2015/01/17. DOI: 10.1038/ni.3054

[48] Blum JS, Wearsch PA, Cresswell P. Pathways of antigen processing. Annual Review of immunology. 2013;**31**:443-473. Epub 2013/01/10. DOI: 10.1146/annurev-immunol-032712-095910

[49] Hogquist KA, Jameson SC, Heath WR, Howard JL, Bevan MJ, Carbone FR. T cell receptor antagonist peptides induce positive selection. Cell. 1994;**76**(1):17-27. Epub 1994/01/14. DOI: 10.1016/0092-8674(94)90169-4

[50] Dimitrov I, Garnev P, Flower DR, Doytchinova I. MHC class II binding prediction-a little help from a friend. Journal of Biomedicine & Biotechnology. 2010;**2010**:705821. Epub 2010/05/29. DOI: 10.1155/2010/705821

[51] Lundegaard C, Lund O, Buus S, Nielsen M. Major histocompatibility complex class I binding predictions as a tool in epitope discovery. Immunology. 2010;**130**(3):309-318. Epub 2010/06/04. DOI: 10.1111/j.1365-2567.2010.03300.x

[52] de Martel C, Georges D, Bray F, Ferlay J, Clifford GM. Global burden of cancer attributable to infections in 2018: A worldwide incidence analysis. The Lancet Global Health. 2020;**8**(2):e180-ee90. Epub 2019/12/22. DOI: 10.1016/s2214-109x(19)30488-7

[53] Schiller JT, Lowy DR. Prospects for preventing cancer with anti-microbial prophylactic vaccines. Cell Host & Microbe. 2023;**31**(1):137-140. Epub 2022/11/25. DOI: 10.1016/j.chom.2022.10.016

[54] Vici P, Pizzuti L, Mariani L, Zampa G, Santini D, Di Lauro L, et al. Targeting immune response with therapeutic vaccines in premalignant lesions and cervical cancer: Hope or reality from clinical studies. Expert Review of Vaccines. 2016;**15**(10):1327-1336. Epub 2016/04/12. DOI: 10.1080/14760584.2016.1176533

[55] Wang N, Chen M, Wang T. Liposomes used as a vaccine adjuvant-delivery system: From basics to clinical immunization. Journal of Controlled Release. 2019;**303**:130-150. Epub 2019/04/26. DOI: 10.1016/j.jconrel.2019.04.025

[56] Kanodia S, Fahey LM, Kast WM. Mechanisms used by human papillomaviruses to escape the host immune response. Current Cancer Drug Targets. 2007;**7**(1):79-89. Epub 2007/02/20. DOI: 10.2174/156800907780006869

[57] Zhong L, Krummenacher C, Zhang W, Hong J, Feng Q, Chen Y, et al. Urgency and necessity of Epstein-Barr virus prophylactic vaccines. NPJ Vaccines. 2022;**7**(1):159. Epub 2022/12/10. DOI: 10.1038/s41541-022-00587-6

[58] Rzymski P, Szuster-Ciesielska A, Dzieciątkowski T, Gwenzi W, Fal A. mRNA vaccines: The future of prevention of viral infections? Journal of Medical Virology. 2023;**95**(2):e28572. Epub 2023/02/11. DOI: 10.1002/jmv.28572

[59] Casper C, Corey L, Cohen JI, Damania B, Gershon AA, Kaslow DC, et al. KSHV (HHV8) vaccine: Promises and potential pitfalls for a new anti-cancer vaccine. NPJ Vaccines. 2022;**7**(1):108. Epub 2022/09/21. DOI: 10.1038/s41541-022-00535-4

[60] Baudino TA. Targeted cancer therapy: The next generation of cancer treatment. Current Drug Discovery Technologies. 2015;**12**(1):3-20. Epub 2015/06/03. DOI: 10.2174/1570163812666150602144310

[61] Imyanitov EN, Iyevleva AG. Molecular tests for prediction of tumor sensitivity to cytotoxic drugs. Cancer Letters. 2022;**526**:41-52. Epub 2021/11/23. DOI: 10.1016/j.canlet.2021.11.021

[62] Gerl R, Vaux DL. Apoptosis in the development and treatment of cancer. Carcinogenesis. 2005;**26**(2):263-270. Epub 2004/09/18. DOI: 10.1093/carcin/bgh283

[63] García-Becerra R, Santos N, Díaz L, Camacho J. Mechanisms of resistance to endocrine therapy in breast cancer: Focus on signaling pathways, miRNAs and genetically based resistance. International Journal of Molecular Sciences. 2012;**14**(1):108-145. Epub 2013/01/25. DOI: 10.3390/ijms14010108

[64] Montagna E, Colleoni M. Hormonal treatment combined with targeted therapies in endocrine-responsive and HER2-positive metastatic breast cancer. Therapeutic Advances in Medical Oncology. 2019;**11**:1758835919894105. Epub 2020/01/04. DOI: 10.1177/1758835919894105

[65] Chen I, Chen MY, Goedegebuure SP, Gillanders WE. Challenges targeting cancer neoantigens in 2021: A systematic literature review. Expert Review of Vaccines. 2021;**20**(7):827-837. Epub 2021/05/29. DOI: 10.1080/14760584.2021.1935248

[66] Asimgil H, Ertetik U, Çevik NC, Ekizce M, Doğruöz A, Gökalp M, et al. Targeting the undruggable oncogenic KRAS: The dawn of hope. JCI Insight. 2022;**7**(1):e153688. Epub 2022/01/12. DOI: 10.1172/jci.insight.153688

[67] Jou J, Harrington KJ, Zocca MB, Ehrnrooth E, Cohen EEW. The changing landscape of therapeutic cancer vaccines-novel platforms and Neoantigen identification. Clinical Cancer Research. 2021;**27**(3):689-703. Epub 2020/10/31. DOI: 10.1158/1078-0432.Ccr-20-0245

[68] Zheng Y, Zhong Z. Roadmap to next-generation cancer vaccines. Journal of Controlled Release. 2022;**347**:308-313. Epub 2022/05/14. DOI: 10.1016/j.jconrel.2022.05.005

[69] Mougel A, Terme M, Tanchot C. Therapeutic cancer vaccine and combinations with antiangiogenic therapies and immune checkpoint blockade. Frontiers in Immunology. 2019;**10**:467. Epub 2019/03/30. DOI: 10.3389/fimmu.2019.00467

Chapter 5

Perspective Chapter: RNA Therapeutics for Cancers

Michiko Kurikawa, Marimu Sakumoto and Akihide Yoshimi

Abstract

RNA therapeutics represent a promising class of drugs and some of the successful therapeutics have been recently transformed into clinics for several disorders. A growing body of evidence has underlined the involvement of aberrant expression of cancer-associate genes or RNA splicing in the pathogenesis of a variety of cancers. In addition, there have been >200 clinical trials of oligonucleotide therapeutics targeting a variety of molecules in cancers. Although there are no approved RNA therapeutics against cancers so far, some promising outcomes have been obtained in phase 1/2 clinical trials. We will review the recent advances in the study of cancer pathogenesis associated with RNA therapeutics and the development of RNA therapeutics for cancers.

Keywords: nucleic acid therapeutics, antisense oligonucleotide, cancer, aptamer, clinical trial

1. Introduction

Nucleic acid plays a central role in biology and it is an attractive tool for therapeutic applications due to multiple reasons. One of the major obstacles is the low *in vivo* stability of nucleic acid therapeutics due to nuclease sensitivity. Numerous synthetic oligonucleotides have been developed to overcome this obstacle using chemical modifications, phosphate backbone, and many other technologies. Some of these technologies have been shown to potently protect the oligonucleotides from degradation and enable efficient cellular uptake, which could be translated into the clinic. In fact, some RNA therapeutics have shown dramatic effects on neurodegenerative disorders such as spinal muscular atrophy and amyotrophic lateral sclerosis. Although there has been no approved RNA therapeutics in oncology so far, researchers have obtained a number of promising results from preclinical and clinical studies. In this chapter, we will concisely summarize the general characteristics of RNA therapeutics and review recent advances in the development of RNA therapeutics in the oncology field.

2. RNA therapeutics

RNA therapeutics represents a therapy with the use of RNA-based molecules to modulate molecular and biological processes to cure a specific disease or improve symptoms. There are multiple classes of RNA therapeutics and each of them has its own strengths which would be difficult to achieve by using other drug modalities.

2.1 Classification of RNA therapeutics

Oligonucleotide therapeutics that have been investigated in clinical trials include antisense oligonucleotides (ASOs), small interfering RNAs (siRNAs), microRNAs (miRNAs) and aptamers (**Figure 1**).

2.1.1 Antisense oligonucleotide (ASO)

ASOs are small (~18–30 nucleotides), synthetic, single-stranded nucleic acid polymers that are complementary to the specific RNA through Watson-Crick base-pairing [1]. They are highly sensitive to degradation by nucleases in their naked form. In addition, their phosphodiester backbone makes it difficult to go through the plasma membrane. To resolve these issues, numerous efforts have been made to improve these situations by chemically modifying ASOs. As a result, there are currently three generations of modified ASOs. Chemical modifications and pharmacological profiles were reviewed in detail elsewhere such as in [2]. The main mechanisms of approved ASOs are classified into the following two categories [3]:

i. ASOs in the first category induce the cleavage of a target mRNA by binding to the target sequence. When this category of ASOs binds to the target mRNA, RNase H endonuclease recognizes the RNA-DNA heteroduplex, degrades the mRNA and downregulates gene expression.

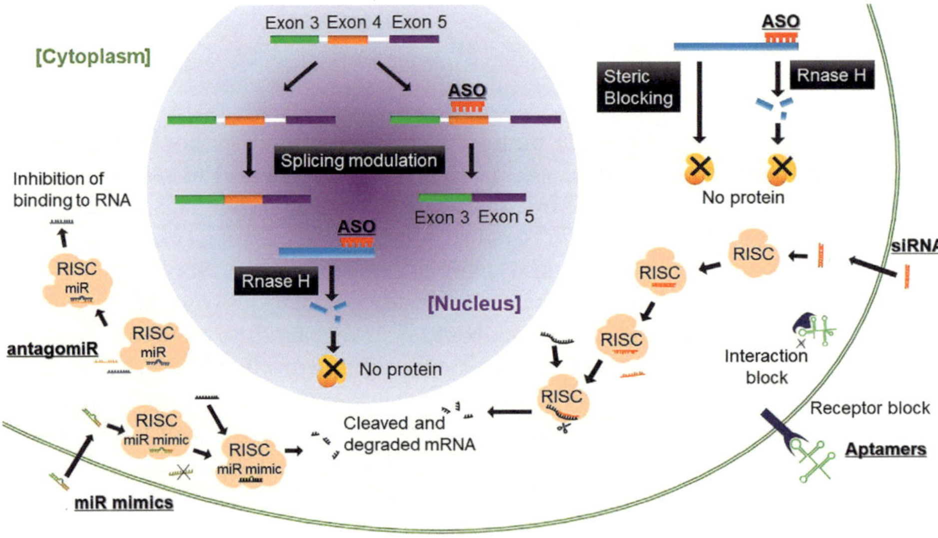

Figure 1.
A variety of RNA therapeutics and their mechanisms. Endocytosis is the main pathway for oligonucleotides to enter cells. Antisense oligonucleotides (ASOs) block the translation of target messenger RNA (mRNA) in RNase H-dependent and -independent manners. ASOs are also able to modulate RNA splicing. Mature mRNA is targeted by small interfering RNAs (siRNAs). The roles of microRNAs (miRNAs) are mainly classified into two types: miRNA mimetics that restore the levels of miRNAs and antagomiRs that suppress expression levels of target miRNA. Aptamers functions to block receptors, protein-protein interactions, etc. like antibodies, but they are smaller in size and easier to pass through the cell membrane compared to antibodies.

ii. ASOs in the second category regulate splicing of pre-mRNAs generally by blocking the binding of splicing factors to cis-element such as splice sites, exonic splicing enhancer (ESE) and intronic splicing silencer (ISS). This category of ASOs is the most widely used strategy.

2.1.2 Small interfering RNA (siRNA)

siRNAs are non-coding RNAs that degrade the mRNA of the targeted gene. Exogenous double-stranded precursor siRNAs are taken up into the cell and processed by Dicer into 20–25 bp long, which are passed to Argonaut (Ago) protein and the sense strand is released [4]. The remaining antisense strand and Ago then form an RNA-induced silencing complex (RISC). Finally, the RISC seeks out and binds to the target mRNA and degrades it [5].

2.1.3 microRNA (miRNA)

In addition to siRNA, miRNA is another RNA therapy based on RNA interference. miRNA is a small non-coding RNA that degrades mRNA in the same way as siRNA. However, its mechanism is slightly different from that of siRNA. Transcripts expressed from miRNA genes are single-stranded RNAs, taking a hairpin structure. In the nucleus, miRNA transcripts undergo primary processing by Dorsha [6], which has an RNase III domain, and after that, Exportin5 transports them to the cytoplasm. In the cytoplasm, miRNAs receive secondary processing by Dicer and are cleaved as double-stranded miRNAs [7]. As with siRNAs, the single-stranded miRNAs then bind to Ago protein and form RISC. In addition, GW182 protein is required for target RNA degradation [8]. Via GW182, some RNA degrading enzymes assemble on the RNA and RISC destabilizes RNA instability.

2.1.4 Aptamers

The other category is RNA therapy targeting proteins. Aptamers are short single-stranded nucleic acids that bind to proteins. Its properties are achieved by its tertiary structures. Aptamer can have a wide range of functions including agonists [9, 10], antagonists [11, 12], bispecific aptamers [13, 14] and carriers for other drugs [15, 16]. Although its function is similar to antibodies, RNA aptamers are smaller in size and easier to pass through the cell membrane.

2.2 Advantages of RNA therapeutics

RNA therapy has several valuable strengths, which make the development of RNA technologies a worthwhile investment. These advantages could be summarized below:

2.2.1 Targeting the untargetable, treating the untreatable

One of the greatest advantages of RNA therapeutics is nicely condensed in the phrase above. RNA drugs can target "undruggable" molecules that are difficult or impossible to target with small molecule-based drugs or other modalities. Only about one-third of proteins can be targeted by common drugs such as small molecules and antibodies [17]. In addition, many proteins share similar structures, which makes it difficult to target specific proteins. On the other hand, as RNA drugs can indirectly act on proteins before the translation, they function independently of protein structure. Furthermore, small molecules and monoclonal antibodies exert their effects by binding to the active site pocket of receptors or enzymes. For this reason, it is impossible for conventional drugs to target non-coding RNAs that are not translated. RNA drugs can target non-coding RNAs and are expected to greatly expand the range of therapeutic targets in the future [3]. We will review some examples of previously "undruggable" targets for which clinical trials are currently ongoing.

2.2.2 Quick production

As we all enjoyed the significant benefits from mRNA vaccines for coronavirus disease-2019 (COVID-19) in recent years, the next important advantage of RNA therapeutics is that RNA drugs can be designed and synthesized rapidly for clinical tests. Given that the development of small molecule or antibody-based drugs takes several years, this characteristic of RNA therapy is the biggest reason that we were able to control the COVID-19 pandemic by significantly reducing the rate of infection and the severity of the disease. By simply changing the sequence of RNA drugs according to the target genes/diseases, researchers can quickly create a novel RNA therapeutic for further testing within a short period of time. This leads to another advantage below.

2.2.3 Patient-customized therapy

Pharmaceutical companies generally hold the back investment for rare diseases as the market is small and the cost-benefit ratio is normally not attractive. However, RNA therapy might be a game changer in this scenario. A landmark trial of patient-customized ASO therapy for neuronal ceroid lipofuscinosis 7 (CLN7), a fatal neurodegenerative disorder (a form of Batten's disease) was reported in 2019 [18]. In this case, a mutation located in intron 6 of MFSD8 creates a novel acceptor, leading to a cryptic exon with a premature stop codon. The authors developed a tailored ASO to rescue the mis-splicing event and delivered it to the patient within 1 year after first contact with the patient. This led to a reduction in seizures without any serious adverse events. The fact that rare diseases affect approximately 30 million persons in the United States alone [19] highlights the importance of such rapid development of patient-customized treatments.

3. Current advances in the development of RNA therapy for cancers

Targeted therapies have greatly improved cancer management by specifically targeting the genetic alterations and consequent molecular disturbances that play an essential role in cancer initiation and maintenance. One of the major therapeutic successes would be inhibitors that specifically target constitutively active tyrosine kinases, such as imatinib and its second- and third-generation inhibitors specifically targeting BCR-ABL against Philadelphia chromosome-positive chronic myeloid leukemia (CML) [20] and acute lymphoblastic leukemia (ALL) [21]. Before the development of imatinib, treatment with interferon alfa plus cytarabine was standard care for patients with CML. In the landmark clinical trial of imatinib, newly diagnosed chronic-phase CML patients were treated with either imatinib or interferon alfa plus cytarabine. After a median follow-up of 19 months, the major cytogenetic response was 87.1% in the imatinib group versus 34.7% in the combination therapy group ($P < 0.001$) [20]. Based on the clearly superior therapeutic outcome, imatinib became the first-line therapy in newly diagnosed chronic-phase CML. Other successful targeted therapies include vemurafenib for the constitutively active form of the BRAF kinase (BRAF^{V600E}) in BRAF-V600E mutated metastatic melanoma [22] and the blocking antibodies such as anti-EGFR antibody for metastatic colon cancer [23] and anti-HER2 antibody for breast cancer with HER-2 amplification) [24].

On the other hand, targeted therapies remained to be developed for many other cancer-associated genes, especially for other 'undruggable' targets such as RAS and MYC. Although there has been no approved RNA therapy for cancers so far, extensive efforts have been focused on targeting such 'undruggable' targets by using a variety of RNA therapeutics, which will be introduced in this section.

3.1 ASO therapy

Targeted therapies through ASO have been most actively studied among RNA therapeutic and approximately half of ongoing clinical trials on RNA therapeutics are classified as this modality. Recently developed ASO therapies against cancers are summarized in **Table 1**.

NCT Number	Phase	RNA therapy	Target	Start date	Status
NCT05267899	Phase 1	Cancers	AKT1	2022/8/1	Not yet recruiting
NCT02144051	Phase 1	Prostate cancer	AR	2014/5/1	Completed
NCT03300505	Phase 1/2	Prostate cancer	AR	2019/5/31	Suspended
NCT04072458	Phase 1	Lymphoid malignancies	BCL2	2020/11/5	Recruiting
NCT04504669	Phase 1	Cancers	FOXP3	2020/8/18	Recruiting
NCT02781883	Phase 2	AML	GRB2	2016/5/1	Recruiting
NCT02923986	Phase 1/2	Ph-ALL	GRB2	2017/9/1	Withdrawn
NCT04196257	Phase 1	Cancers	GRB2	2022/7/1	Not yet recruiting
NCT01780545	Phase 2	Bladder cancer	HSP27	2013/4/1	Completed
NCT02423590	Phase 2	Squamous cell lung cancers	HSP27	2014/6/1	Unknown status
NCT04485949	Phase 2	Glioblastoma	IFG-1R	2022/12/1	Not yet recruiting
NCT03101839	Phase 1	Cancers	KRAS	2017/5/15	Completed
NCT01563302	Phase 1/2	Cancers	STAT3	2012/2/27	Completed
NCT01839604	Phase 1	Hepatocellular carcinoma	STAT3	2013/5/1	Completed
NCT02417753	Phase 2	Cancers	STAT3	2015/4/3	Terminated
NCT02549651	Phase 1	DLBCL	STAT3	2016/7/13	Completed
NCT04862767	Phase 1	Cancers	TGF-β2	2021/3/9	Recruiting
NCT02243124	Phase 1	MDS	TP53	2014/9/1	Terminated

Abbreviations: AR, androgen receptor; AML, acute myeloid leukemia; Ph-ALL, Philadelphia-chromosome positive acute lymphoblastic leukemia; DLBCL, diffuse large B-cell lymphoma; MDS, myelodysplastic syndromes. *The table does not include all the recent clinical trials on ASO therapies in oncology. This equally applies to* **Tables 2–4**.

Table 1.
*Recent ASO therapy in clinical trials.**

Some of the landmark trials in this field were performed or are currently performed as follows:

3.1.1 ASO therapy against MYB

Historically, the first clinical trial of ASO in oncology was a phase II study back in 1993, which evaluated G4460, an ASO targeting MYB in CML (NCT00002592). *MYB* is a proto-oncogene that encode a transcription factor. As evidenced by the discovery of translocations and duplications of *MYB* in a subset of T-cell acute lymphoblastic leukemia (T-ALL) [25, 26], MYB activation was shown to contribute to the leukemogenesis via differentiation block [25]. In addition, early studies using an antisense oligodeoxynucleotide and dominant-negative form of MYB have demonstrated that MYB activation is important for the proliferative capacity of myeloid malignancies such as AML and CML. Another study indicated that an oligomer complementary to the sequence of *MYB*-encoded mRNA resulted in significant growth inhibition in several leukemic cell lines [27, 28]. Based on these observations, G4460 was designed to bind the MYB mRNA and trigger RNase H-dependent degradation [29]. In a pilot study, $CD34^+$ marrow autografts were purged with G4460 in allograft-ineligible CML patients. Although the clinical efficacy of G4460 could not be assessed in this pilot study, MYB mRNA levels were significantly reduced in approximately 50% of patients, suggesting the feasibility of transplanting G4460-treated autografts [29]. As described above, the standard treatment strategy for CML has been dramatically changed since imatinib and other tyrosine kinase inhibitors were developed. Nonetheless, MYB is an attractive target, considering that overexpression of MYB is associated with cellular proliferation and differentiation in multiple cancers including several types of leukemias and breast cancers [30].

3.1.2 ASO therapy targeting BCL2

BCL2 family of proteins have long been identified for their roles in apoptosis. BCL2 was initially discovered in the context of B-cell lymphoma in the 1980s, followed by the identification of a variety of homologous proteins [31–33]. The role of the BCL2 family is typically understood as the anti-apoptotic and pro-apoptotic members. By regulating outer mitochondrial membrane (OMM) integrity and function, BCL2 facilitates oncogenesis through cell death resistance [34]. In cancer, increased expression of BCL2 protein is frequently found [35] and is commonly associated with reduced susceptibility to chemotherapy and increased radioresistance [36]. These observations provided a rationale to target BCL2 in a variety of cancers.

Genasense (oblimersen, G3139) would be a representative ASO targeting BCL2, which targets codon 1–6 of BCL2 mRNA and triggers RNase H-dependent degradation [37]. More than 40 clinical trials have been performed on this ASO in a variety of types of cancers and Genasense obtained orphan drug designation for CLL in 2001. However, overall and progression-free survival was not affected and the primary endpoint was not reached by the treatment of Genasense in the following eight phase III studies. For example, combined fludarabine + cyclophosphamide + Genasense therapy resulted in a better response (complete + partial response) rate over fludarabine + cyclophosphamide therapy in CLL, which fulfilled only the second endpoint of the NCT00024440 trial [38]. Following these unsatisfactory results, Genasense was not approved and the production of Genasense was ceased.

Several other ASOs such as SPC2996 and PNT2258 have been developed to target BCL2. SPC2996 is a gapmer that targets the first six codons of the BCL2 mRNA. Although the phase 1/2 trial for evaluating SPC2996 was performed in CLL, approximately 40% of patients experienced painful inflammatory reactions [39]. PNT2258 is a liposome-encapsulated ASO that targets the BCL2 promoter to suppress its transcription. Although the safety of PNT2258 was confirmed in the phase 1 study, the following phase 2 trial targeting patients with diffuse large B-cell lymphoma (DLBCL) resulted in an unsatisfactory outcome with a very low response rate of 8.1%.

Following these failures of ASOs targeting BCL2, the development of ASOs against BCL2 slowed down. In 2016, the selective BCL2 inhibitor ABT-199 (venetoclax), a BH3 mimetic was approved as the first small molecule drug targeting a protein-protein interaction for chronic lymphocytic leukemia (CLL) [40]. Venetoclax has been also approved for the treatment of AML in combination with other chemotherapeutic agents such as DNA demethylating agents and low-dose cytarabine [41].

3.1.3 ASO therapy targeting IFG-1R

Results from a unique clinical study were reported in 2021 [42]. In this phase IB clinical trial, the safety and efficacy of IMV-001, an antisense oligodeoxynucleotide against IGF type 1 receptor (IGF-1R) mRNA were evaluated in adults with newly diagnosed glioblastoma. Glioblastoma is one of the most aggressive forms of brain cancer which represents approximately 15% of all brain tumors [43]. Despite intensive treatment, glioblastoma almost always recurs, leading to a dismal prognosis with a median survival of 10–13 months [44]. On the other hand, IFG-1R is highly expressed in a variety of malignancies, which regulates transformation and anti-apoptotic effects and are essential for the survival and progression of malignant cells [45–48]. However, previous efforts to target IGF-1R alone were not successful [48]. Interestingly, IMV-001 had an off-target effect to activate Toll-like receptor 9 (TLR9) in antigen-presenting cells [49, 50], which stimulates the immune response. Therefore, the research group from Thomas Jefferson University designed a phase IA trial of IGV-001 to use an autologous cell combination product therapy [51]. More specifically, 12 patients underwent MRI-based image-guided tumor resection (which resulted in partial resections in all the cases). After diagnostic confirmation, an abdominal acceptor site between the rectus sheath and rectus abdominis muscle was created. On the other hand, the resected tumor cells were treated with IMV-001 *ex vivo* and encapsulated in several chambers. Immediately after irradiation to the tumor cells, chambers were implanted in the acceptor site and removed after 24 h (**Figure 2**).

While 3 of 12 patients were re-treated after the approval from FDA was obtained, 8 patients received no other treatment except surgical resection and/or best support care (and the other one exceptional case received temozolomide). As a result, there were no unexpected treatment-related complications except deep vein thrombosis, which was successfully managed by enoxaparin prophylaxis. Post-treatment observation identified two and four patients with complete and partial responses, respectively, which were atypical for the nature of aggressive glioblastoma. Among the patients with these responses with disease recurrence, three patients had unusual regression spontaneously or after surgical resection. Interestingly, perivascular lymphocytic infiltration was observed in some patients who did not have such infiltration at diagnosis, strongly suggesting a contribution of the immune response. Based on these results, IGV-001 was granted Orphan Drug designation by FDA in 2017. A total 33 newly diagnosed patients with glioblastoma were enrolled in the subsequent Phase

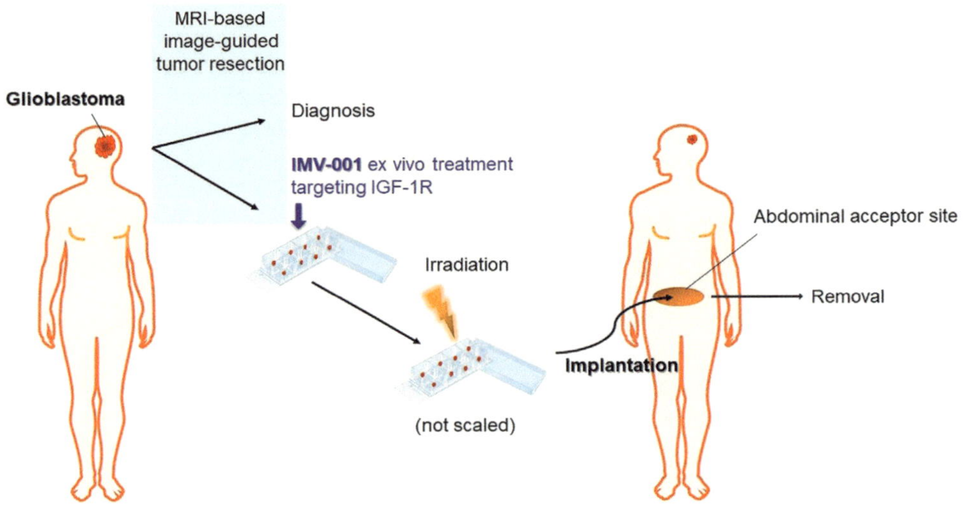

Figure 2.
Study design for the IGV-001 treatment. After MRI-based image-guided tumor resection and diagnostic confirmation, an abdominal acceptor site between the rectus sheath and rectus abdominis muscle was created. The resected tumor cells were treated with IMV-001 ex vivo and encapsulated in several chambers. Immediately after irradiation to the tumor cells, chambers were implanted in the acceptor site and removed.

IB study (ClinicalTrials.gov: NCT02507583). In this study, patients received IGV-001 and standard care which consists of maximal safe resection, adjuvant radiotherapy and temozolomide and maintenance therapy with temozolomide. Median progression-free survival (PFS) in the intent-to-treat population was 9.8 months, which was significantly better than that of patients who received standard care in published studies (6.5 months; P = 0.0003). Because the promoter methylation status of the *MGMT* gene was previously shown to positively predict the therapeutic efficacy of temozolomide [52, 53] and overall survival (OS) [54], the authors quantified the methylation levels of *MGMT* and revealed that the *MGMT* methylation status is a potent biomarker for PFS and OS. Furthermore, they assessed serum cytokines and identified that some of the pro-inflammatory cytokines such as IFNγ and IL-2 were elevated after IGV-001 treatment (before initiation of standard care). Although these responses were not associated with therapeutic outcomes, these results suggested that IGV-001 treatment induces a local environment at implantation which promotes a proinflammatory innate immune response [42].

3.2 siRNA therapy

Although most clinical trials on siRNA drugs in oncology are currently phase 1, there are some promising results from these trials. In addition, some phase 2 trials have been recently initiated (**Table 2**).

3.2.1 siRNA therapy targeting MYC

MYC is one of the most famous and most commonly activated oncogenes and has thus far been considered one of the major "undruggable" targets in cancers. As described above, a therapeutic approach using RNA interference (siRNA) is a

NCT Number	Phase	RNA therapy	Target	Start date	Status
NCT04844983	Phase 2	cSCC	TGF-β1 and COX2	2021/5/18	Recruiting
NCT02866916	Phase 1	Prostate cancer	AR	2017/9/1	Withdrawn
NCT02166255	Phase 1	Cancers	CBLB	2014/12/1	Completed
NCT03087591	Phase 1	Cancers	CBLB	2017/4/28	Completed
NCT01591356	Phase 1	Cancers	EPHA2	2015/7/1	Recruiting
NCT03819387	Phase 1	Cancers	GST	2019/3/18	Recruiting
NCT01676259	Phase 2	Pancreatic cancer	KRASG12D	2018/3/7	Recruiting
NCT03608631	Phase 1	Pancreatic cancer	KRASG12D	2021/1/27	Recruiting
NCT02110563	Phase 1	Cancers	MYC	2014/4/1	Terminated
NCT02314052	Phase 1/2	Hepatocellular carcinoma	MYC	2015/1/27	Terminated
NCT01808638	Phase 1/2	Pancreatic cancer	PNK3	2013/3/1	Completed
NCT04995536	Phase 1	NHL	STAT3	2022/8/1	Recruiting

Abbreviations: cSCC, cutaneous squamous cell carcinoma; NHL, non-Hodgkin lymphoma.

Table 2.
Recent siRNA therapy in clinical trials.

promising strategy because a number of studies have shown that silencing MYC induces growth inhibition in MYC-activated tumors in multiple cellular and animal models. An anti-MYC siRNA formulated in lipid nanoparticles called DCR-MYC has shown anti-tumor potential *in vivo* across several tumor models [55]. In phase 1 dose-escalation study, 19 patients with a variety of cancers were treated with DCR-MYC. DCR-MYC was well tolerated and demonstrated promising clinical efficacy across various dose levels, including a complete response in one patient and tumor regression in several other patients, validating the hypothesis that siRNA targeting *MYC* is a potential therapeutic strategy to make the "undruggable" target druggable.

Recently, another strategy to pharmacologically target MYC was reported [56]. In this study, the authors performed a pan-cancer transcriptome and splicing analysis of RNA sequence data generated from cancer patients with or without hotspot mutations in *SF3B1*, which is the most frequently mutated splicing factor across cancer [57, 58]. In this study, detailed molecular and biological experiments using isogenic murine models and cancer patient samples revealed that a mis-splicing event in *PPP2R5A* induces MYC activation via post-translational modifications. More specifically, mutant SF3B1 induced 3′ alternative splice site in *PPP2R5A*, which led to a reduced protein expression of PPP2R5A, a regulatory B subunit of PP2A phosphatase complex. PP2A complex containing PPP2R5A was shown to regulate phosphorylation of MYC protein which was critical for the regulation of protein stability. Therefore, loss of PPP2R5A function stabilized MYC protein. Importantly, FDA-approved activator FTY-720 suppressed mutant SF3B1 leukemogenesis *in vivo*, providing a preclinical insight into the use of PP2A activators in SF3B1 mutant cancers [56]. Furthermore, the mis-splicing event in *PPP2R5A* can be potentially targeted by a specific ASO, which will also create a therapeutic opportunity for pharmacological intervention toward activated MYC.

3.2.2 siRNA therapy targeting mutant KRAS

Another "undruggable" target commonly detected across cancers, especially in pancreatic cancers is a hotspot mutation in *KRAS*. Based on the results that siRNA-mediated KRAS silencing resulted in growth inhibition of pancreatic cancer cells *in vitro* and *in vivo*, Silenseed Ltd. has developed a siRNA drug named siG12D-LODER, which is a siRNA targeting KRAS G12D and other additional G12X mutations such as G12C and G12V with a miniature biodegradable polymeric matrix. LODER™ allows slow and prolonged local release of the encapsulated drug. siG12D-LODER was designed to keep releasing the drug for 4 months, which can be inserted into the pancreatic tumor via a standard endoscope ultrasound-guided biopsy procedure.

In the phase 1/2a dose escalation and expansion study, patients with pancreatic cancer received a one-time dose of siG12D-LODER via endoscopic intervention with chemotherapy including gemcitabine or FOLFIRINOX. The combination of chemotherapy and siG12D-LODER was safe and well-tolerated, with five of 15 treated patients experiencing serious adverse events including grade 3–4 neutropenia and cholangitis. Regarding efficacy, the median OS was 15.1 months. Tumor progression was not observed in any patients at 8 weeks after the treatment. In addition, in 10 patients whose tumor marker CA19-9 levels were elevated at enrollment, more than 20% decrease in CA19-9 levels were observed in seven patients [59]. Following these promising results, a phase 2 clinical trial is recruiting patients with both borderline resectable and locally advanced pancreatic cancer [60].

3.3 miRNA therapy

Compared to the ASO and siRNA modalities, the number of clinical trials for evaluating miRNA therapeutics is limited as below (**Table 3**). However, research on miRNA or miRNA therapeutics are being greatly increased in number, according to a survey by Bonneau et al. [61].

Here are some examples of miRNA therapeutics developed or being developed. Therapeutic strategies using miRNA are mainly classified into the following two groups: (1) AntagomiRs to repress overexpressed miRNAs (Example: MRG-106), and (2) miRNA mimetics to restore downregulated miRNAs (Example: MRX34).

NCT number	Phase	RNA therapy	Target	Start date	Status
NCT04675996	Phase 1	Cancers	JNK1	2020/12/18	Recruiting
NCT03713320	Phase 2	CTCL	miR-155	2019/4/2	Terminated
NCT03837457	Phase 2	CTCL	miR-155	2019/10/1	Terminated
NCT01829971	Phase 1	Cancers	miR-34a	2013/4/1	Terminated
NCT02862145	Phase 1/2	Melanoma	miR-34a	2016/8/1	Withdrawn
NCT02369198	Phase 1	Cancers	miR-16	2014/9/1	Completed

Abbreviation: CTCL, cutaneous T-cell lymphoma cutaneous squamous cell carcinoma.

Table 3.
Recent miRNA therapy in clinical trials.

3.3.1 miRNA therapy against miR-155

miR-155 is overexpressed in various malignancies, especially in cutaneous T-cell lymphoma (CTCL) including Mycosis fungoides (MF) [62–64], and is associated with enhanced cell proliferation and survival [65–67] and genomic instability [68, 69]. In addition, in a number of studies, genetically engineered mice with overexpression of miR-155 murine homolog in lymphoid cells had an increased susceptibility to develop lymphomas and leukemias [64, 70–72]. Molecularly, miR-155 directly targets SHIP1 [73], SOCS1 [74] and some other cancer-associated genes. Overexpression of miR-155 is also related to activation of the PI3K-AKT [75], NF-κB [76] and JAK/STAT [77] pathways. Collectively, these observations provided a rationale to target miR-155 in cancer therapy.

Evidenced by these scientific results, miRagen therapeutics has developed cobomarsen (MRG-106), an oligonucleotide inhibitor of miR-155 which is optimized for efficient uptake in $CD4^+$ T-cell and MF cells with lipid nanoparticles. Cobomarsen was shown to de-repress direct miR-155 target genes as well as de-activate multiple survival pathways in MF cell lines *in vitro* [78]. The phase 1 trial of cobomarsen recruited 15 patients with biopsy-proven stage I-III MF [79]. Intratumoral or subcutaneous administration of cobomarsen resulted in almost no clinically significant adverse events. On the other hand, histological examination of pre- and post-treatment tissue revealed a reduction in cell density and depth in most patients. In addition, a gene expression analysis on these specimens demonstrated significant inactivation of PI3K-AKT, NF-κB and JAK/STAT pathways. This led to the Orphan Drug Designation of cobomarsen for MF type CTCL in 2017 and the initiation of phase 2 trials.

3.3.2 miR-34a based therapeutic

Accumulating evidence has demonstrated the presence of a normally small fraction of cancer cells, cancer stem cells (CSCs) which share stem-like properties with normal stem cells such as self-renewal and differentiation capacities. miR-34 is a tumor suppressive miRNA whose expression is frequently downregulated in many cancers [80] and CSCs.

miR-34 family is one of the three major tumor suppressive miRNA families consisting of miR-34a, miR-34b and miR-34c. Among them, miR-34a is known to repress the expression of >200 target genes and loss of miR-34a biologically regulates tumor growth by inhibiting multiple processes such as cell cycle, epithelial-to-mesenchymal transition, metastasis, immune response and stemness [81–83].

In addition, the loss of miR-34a is associated with CSC regulation in multiple cancer types. For example, MET, NOTCH1 and NOTCH2 were identified as direct targets of miR-34a in glioma stem cells [84] and restoration of miR-34a expression induced differentiation of glioma stem cells with increased expression of astrocyte and oligodendrocyte markers [85]. Another example comes from colorectal cancer where miR-34a functions as a cell-fate determinant of CSCs in this malignancy. Bu et al. identified that high miR-34a expression decreased both symmetric and asymmetric division (resulting in decreased CSCs and increased more differentiated daughter cells), while low miR-34a expression enhanced symmetric CSC-CSC division and suppressed asymmetric division [86].

The first-in-human phase 1 study was initiated to evaluate the maximum tolerated dose, safety, pharmacokinetics and clinical activity of MRX34, a liposomal miR-34a mimic in 47 patients with advanced tumors [87]. Although MRX34 demonstrated some clinical response, including one patient with hepatocellular carcinoma exhibiting a prolonged partial response for 48 weeks and four patients with stable disease for more than 16 weeks, the trial was halted by FDA in 2016 due to severe immune reactions and deaths in four patients in the expansion cohort.

3.4 Aptamer therapy

Although there are only a limited number of clinical trials for Aptamer therapy as is miRNA therapeutics (**Table 4**), there are some promising results, especially from the studies on the aptamer targeting CXCL12.

3.4.1 Aptamer therapy targeting CXCL12

CLL is the most common adult form of leukemia in Western countries which is characterized by the expansion of mature monoclonal B-cells. It has been known that the tissue microenvironment confers survival advantage and drug resistance to the CLL cells via CXC chemokine ligand CXCL12 and other factors such as BAFF, APRIL and CD40 ligand [88–90]. Therefore, drug development has been focused on strategies that interrupt the crosstalk between CCL cells and the stroma such as bone marrow (BM) stroma cells (BMSCs). Importantly, the migration of CLL cells in the tissues is controlled by tissue gradients of chemokines. In the BM, CLL cells are attracted by the CXCL12, which is continuously secreted from BMSCs. The close proximity between CLL cells and BMSCs protects CLL cells from spontaneous- and drug-induced

NCT number	Phase	RNA therapy	Target	Start date	Status
NCT03385148	Early Phase 1	Colorectal cancer	PTK7	2017/1/1	Unknown status
NCT01034410	Phase 2	AML	Nucleolin	2010/1/1	Terminated
NCT00881244	Phase 1	Cancers	Nucleolin	2003/9/1	Completed
NCT00740441	Phase 2	Renal cell carcinoma	Nucleolin	2008/8/1	Unknown status
NCT00512083	Phase 2	Leukemia	Nucleolin	2007/7/1	Completed
NCT01486797	Phase 2	CLL	CXCL12	2012/3/1	Completed
NCT01521533	Phase 2	MM	CXCL12	2012/3/1	Completed
NCT01194934	Phase 1	HSCT	CXCL12	2010/8/1	Completed
NCT00976378	Phase 1	HSCT	CXCL12	2009/10/1	Completed
NCT04121455	Phase 1/2	Glioblastoma	CXCL12	2019/9/12	Recruiting
NCT03168139	Phase 1/2	Cancers	CXCL12	2017/4/18	Completed
NCT04901741	Phase 2	Pancreatic Cancer	CXCL12	2022/12/1	Not yet recruiting

Abbreviations: AML, acute myeloid leukemia; CLL, chronic lymphocytic leukemia; MM, multiple myeloma; HSCT, hematopoietic stem cell transplantation.

Table 4.
Recent aptamer therapy in clinical trials.

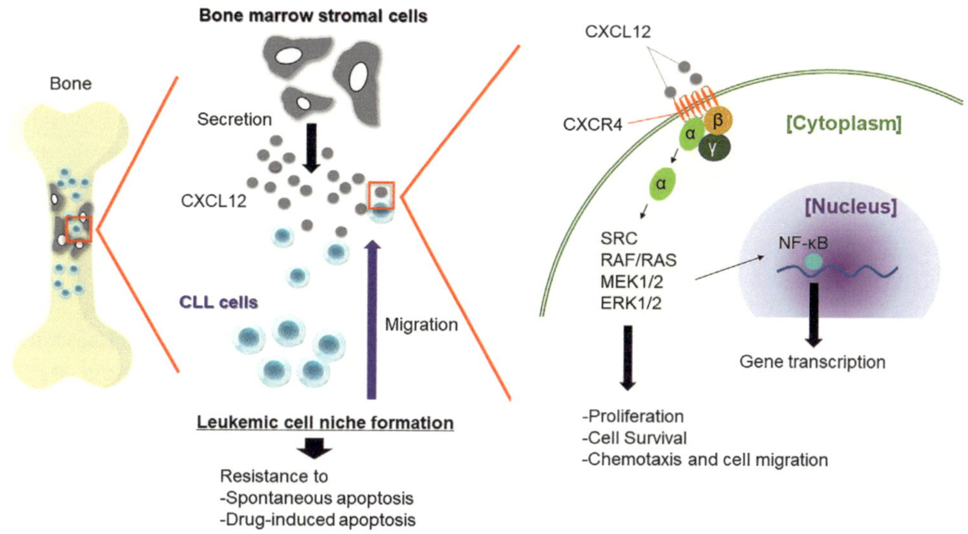

Figure 3.
Schema representing the roles of the CXCL12-CXCR4 axis in CLL. Constitutively secreted CXCL12 from the bone marrow stromal cells attract CLL cells via the chemokine receptor CXCR4, which creates leukemic niche in the bone marrow. Molecularly, CXCR4 activates the downstream multiple cancer-associated pathways such as PII3K/AKT/mTOR, RAS/RAF/MEK/ERK and NF-κB pathways.

apoptosis [90–93]. Besides these protective effects, CXCL12 enhances the expansion of BMSC-dependent pre-B cell clones [94] as well as activates multiple pro-survival pathways associated with ERK1/2, STAT3 and AKT (**Figure 3**) [90, 95, 96].

Because CLL cells are attracted via CXCR4, the chemokine receptor of CXCL12, the first small molecule targeting the CXCL12-CXCR4 axis was developed. A multicenter phase 1 study of plerixafor in combination with the anti-C20 antibody rituximab was performed in 24 patients with relapsed/refractory CLL. In this study, a median 3.3-fold increase of CLL cells in the peripheral blood was observed after the first administration of plerixafor, strongly supporting the mobilizing capacity of the drug on CLL cells or the CXCL12-CXCR4 axis and suggesting that plerixafor would contribute to the sensitization of CLL cells [97].

Another therapeutic approach to target the CXCL12-CXCR4 axis is the blockade of CXCL12. However, CXCL12 is highly evolutionary conserved, which hinders the development of antibody-based drug development for CXCL12. NOX-A12 (Spiegelmer), an RNA oligonucleotide successfully bypassed this issue by using a mirror image configuration of naturally occurring RNA. More specifically, the Spiegelmer technology enables an RNA oligonucleotide to bind target molecules with high affinity and specificity [98, 99]. The major merits of using a mirror-image configuration would be summarized as follows: (i) Spiegelmer is resistant to degradation by nucleases, (ii) Spiegelmer does not hybridize with native nucleic acids, (iii) Spiegelmer is immunologically "cold". NOX-A12 is a Spiegelmer that was designed to bind and antagonize CLCX12.

After a phase 1 trial in healthy volunteers was completed, two clinical trials were initiated. In a phase 1/2 trial (NCT01486797) [100], 28 patients with relapsed/refractory CLL were treated with NOX-A12 (olaptesed pegol) in combination with bendamustine and rituximab (BR). NOX-A12 was well-tolerated and there was no additional toxicity when patients were treated in combination with chemoimmunotherapy. In addition, an overall response rate of 8%, including a complete response of 11% was obtained, with a median PFS of 15.4 months and a 3-year OS of >80%. These results compare favorably with those reported by BR alone and other recent BR combination trials [100–102], warranting further clinical development.

Similarly, NOX-A12 was evaluated in 28 patients with relapsed/refractory multiple myeloma (MM) in phase 2 clinical trial (NCT01521533) [103]. This was based on the scientific observations that CXCL12 plays an essential role in supporting myeloma cells in the bone marrow microenvironment and in mobilizing myeloma cells to the peripheral [104, 105]. Patients with MM were treated with NOX-A12 alone for 2 weeks in the pilot phase, followed by the combination treatment (NOX-A12 + bortezomib and dexamethasone) for up to 8 cycles. There were no unexpected adverse events. The overall response rate was 68%, including a complete response of 7% and a very good partial response of 18%. The median PFS and OS were 7.2 months and 28.3 months, respectively. Given that overall response rates in the previous MM studies of bortezomib and bortezomib-based combination treatment for relapsed/refractory MM patients were mostly within the range of 43–63% [106–111], the outcome of this phase 2 study is favorable. In addition, the overall response rates of CXCR4 inhibitor ulociplumab or plerixafor with bortezomib + dexamethasone were 40% and 51%, respectively [112, 113], suggesting that NOX-A12 is a promising approach to target the CXCL12-CXCR4 axis in MM. The results of these clinical trials emphasize the importance of further evaluation of NOX-A12 in MM.

4. Conclusion

Numerous efforts to develop RNA therapeutics against cancers have been made as we partly introduced in this chapter. Although there is currently no approval of RNA therapeutics in oncology, some of the phase 2 studies yielded promising results, which greatly encourages investigators in the field. On the other hand, oligonucleotide drug delivery has now almost matured to the position of clinical utility (there are excellent reviews on this topic such as [39, 114]). Therefore, it is possible that the outcome of a previously failed oligonucleotide therapeutic could be improved with the use of next-generation oligonucleotide or with a novel drug delivery system. These developments would provide expectation that RNA therapy for many cancers will be soon available through the use of precision genetic medicine.

Acknowledgements

This study is partly supported by the following grants awarded to A.Y.: Science and Technology Platform Program for Advanced Biological Medicine (grant number JP22am0401007) and the Japan-Canada Joint call for Strategic International Collaborative Research Program (SICORP; grant number JP22jm0210085) from the Japan Agency for Medical Research and Development (AMED), Grant-in-Aid for Scientific Research (A) (grant number 21H04828) and Home-Returning Researcher Development Research (grant number 19 K24691) from the Japan Society for the Promotion of Science (JSPS), Fusion Oriented Research for disruptive Science and Technology from Japan Science and Technology Agency (JST) (grant number 22-221036124), National Cancer Center Research and Development Funds (grant number 2020-A-2), ASH Global Research Award from American Society of Hematology (ASH), CDP Special Fellow Achievement Award from Leukemia and Lymphoma Society (LLS), and grants from Shimadzu Science Foundation, The Yasuda Medical Foundation, the Chemo-Sero-Therapeutic Research Institute, The Sumitomo Foundation, the Uehara Memorial Foundation, Princess Takamatsu Cancer Research Fund, Takeda Science Foundation, Mochida Memorial Foundation for Medical and Pharmaceutical Research and Astellas Foundation for Research on Metabolic Disorders.

Author contributions

A.Y. designed the manuscript. M.K., M.S. and A.Y. wrote the manuscript. M.S. and A.Y. prepared all the figures and tables.

Conflict of interest

The authors declare no conflict of interest.

Author details

Michiko Kurikawa, Marimu Sakumoto and Akihide Yoshimi*
Division of Cancer RNA Research, National Cancer Center Research Institute, Tokyo, Japan

*Address all correspondence to: ayoshimi@ncc.go.jp

References

[1] Quemener AM, Bachelot L, Forestier A, Donnou-Fournet E, Gilot D, Galibert MD. The powerful world of antisense oligonucleotides: From bench to bedside. Wiley Interdiscip Reviews RNA. 2020;**11**(5):e1594

[2] Xiong H, Veedu RN, Diermeier SD. Recent advances in oligonucleotide therapeutics in oncology. International Journal of Molecular Sciences. 2021;**22**(7):3295

[3] Kim YK. RNA therapy: Rich history, various applications and unlimited future prospects. Experimental & Molecular Medicine. 2022;**54**(4):455-465

[4] Song JJ, Smith SK, Hannon GJ, Joshua-Tor L. Crystal structure of Argonaute and its implications for RISC slicer activity. Science. 2004;**305**(5689):1434-1437

[5] Wittrup A, Lieberman J. Knocking down disease: A progress report on siRNA therapeutics. Nature Reviews. Genetics. 2015;**16**(9):543-552

[6] Ha M, Kim VN. Regulation of microRNA biogenesis. Nature Reviews. Molecular Cell Biology. 2014;**15**(8):509-524

[7] Lam JK, Chow MY, Zhang Y, Leung SW. siRNA versus miRNA as therapeutics for gene silencing. Molecular Therapy Nucleic Acids. 2015;**4**:e252

[8] Eulalio A, Huntzinger E, Izaurralde E. GW182 interaction with Argonaute is essential for miRNA-mediated translational repression and mRNA decay. Nature Structural & Molecular Biology. 2008;**15**(4):346-353

[9] McNamara JO, Kolonias D, Pastor F, Mittler RS, Chen L, Giangrande PH, et al. Multivalent 4-1BB binding aptamers costimulate CD8+ T cells and inhibit tumor growth in mice. The Journal of Clinical Investigation. 2008;**118**(1):376-386

[10] Dollins CM, Nair S, Boczkowski D, Lee J, Layzer JM, Gilboa E, et al. Assembling OX40 aptamers on a molecular scaffold to create a receptor-activating aptamer. Chemistry & Biology. 2008;**15**(7):675-682

[11] Berezhnoy A, Stewart CA, McNamara JO 2nd, Thiel W, Giangrande P, Trinchieri G, et al. Isolation and optimization of murine IL-10 receptor blocking oligonucleotide aptamers using high-throughput sequencing. Molecular Therapy. 2012;**20**(6):1242-1250

[12] Santulli-Marotto S, Nair SK, Rusconi C, Sullenger B, Gilboa E. Multivalent RNA aptamers that inhibit CTLA-4 and enhance tumor immunity. Cancer Research. 2003;**63**(21):7483-7489

[13] Schrand B, Verma B, Levay A, Patel S, Castro I, Benaduce AP, et al. Radiation-induced enhancement of antitumor T-cell immunity by VEGF-targeted 4-1BB costimulation. Cancer Research. 2017;**77**(6):1310-1321

[14] Schrand B, Berezhnoy A, Brenneman R, Williams A, Levay A, Kong LY, et al. Targeting 4-1BB costimulation to the tumor stroma with bispecific aptamer conjugates enhances the therapeutic index of tumor immunotherapy. Cancer Immunology Research. 2014;**2**(9):867-877

[15] Lozano T, Soldevilla MM, Casares N, Villanueva H, Bendandi M, Lasarte JJ, et al. Targeting inhibition of Foxp3

by a CD28 2'-Fluro oligonucleotide aptamer conjugated to P60-peptide enhances active cancer immunotherapy. Biomaterials. 2016;**91**:73-80

[16] McNamara JO 2nd, Andrechek ER, Wang Y, Viles KD, Rempel RE, Gilboa E, et al. Cell type-specific delivery of siRNAs with aptamer-siRNA chimeras. Nature Biotechnology. 2006;**24**(8):1005-1015

[17] Fauman EB, Rai BK, Huang ES. Structure-based druggability assessment-identifying suitable targets for small molecule therapeutics. Current Opinion in Chemical Biology. 2011;**15**(4):463-468

[18] Kim J, Hu C, Moufawad El Achkar C, Black LE, Douville J, Larson A, et al. Patient-customized oligonucleotide therapy for a rare genetic disease. The New England Journal of Medicine. 2019;**381**(17):1644-1652

[19] Griggs RC, Batshaw M, Dunkle M, Gopal-Srivastava R, Kaye E, Krischer J, et al. Clinical research for rare disease: Opportunities, challenges, and solutions. Molecular Genetics and Metabolism. 2009;**96**(1):20-26

[20] O'Brien SG, Guilhot F, Larson RA, Gathmann I, Baccarani M, Cervantes F, et al. Imatinib compared with interferon and low-dose cytarabine for newly diagnosed chronic-phase chronic myeloid leukemia. The New England Journal of Medicine. 2003;**348**(11):994-1004

[21] Thomas DA, Faderl S, Cortes J, O'Brien S, Giles FJ, Kornblau SM, et al. Treatment of Philadelphia chromosome-positive acute lymphocytic leukemia with hyper-CVAD and imatinib mesylate. Blood. 2004;**103**(12):4396-4407

[22] Chapman PB, Hauschild A, Robert C, Haanen JB, Ascierto P, Larkin J, et al. Improved survival with vemurafenib in melanoma with BRAF V600E mutation. The New England Journal of Medicine. 2011;**364**(26):2507-2516

[23] Li D, Fu Q, Li M, Li J, Yin C, Zhao J, et al. Primary tumor site and anti-EGFR monoclonal antibody benefit in metastatic colorectal cancer: A meta-analysis. Future Oncology. 2017;**13**(12):1115-1127

[24] Ross JS, Slodkowska EA, Symmans WF, Pusztai L, Ravdin PM, Hortobagyi GN. The HER-2 receptor and breast cancer: Ten years of targeted anti-HER-2 therapy and personalized medicine. The Oncologist. 2009;**14**(4):320-368

[25] Clappier E, Cuccuini W, Kalota A, Crinquette A, Cayuela JM, Dik WA, et al. The C-MYB locus is involved in chromosomal translocation and genomic duplications in human T-cell acute leukemia (T-ALL), the translocation defining a new T-ALL subtype in very young children. Blood. 2007;**110**(4):1251-1261

[26] Lahortiga I, De Keersmaecker K, Van Vlierberghe P, Graux C, Cauwelier B, Lambert F, et al. Duplication of the MYB oncogene in T cell acute lymphoblastic leukemia. Nature Genetics. 2007;**39**(5):593-595

[27] Tondelli L, Ricca A, Laus M, Lelli M, Citro G. Highly efficient cellular uptake of c-myb antisense oligonucleotides through specifically designed polymeric nanospheres. Nucleic Acids Research. 1998;**26**(23):5425-5431

[28] Anfossi G, Gewirtz AM, Calabretta B. An oligomer complementary to c-myb-encoded mRNA inhibits proliferation of human myeloid leukemia cell lines. Proceedings of the National Academy of Sciences of the United States of America. 1989;**86**(9):3379-3383

[29] Luger SM, O'Brien SG, Ratajczak J, Ratajczak MZ, Mick R, Stadtmauer EA, et al. Oligodeoxynucleotide-mediated inhibition of c-myb gene expression in autografted bone marrow: A pilot study. Blood. 2002;**99**(4):1150-1158

[30] Fry EA, Inoue K. c-MYB and DMTF1 in cancer. Cancer Investigation. 2019;**37**(1):46-65

[31] Tsujimoto Y. Stress-resistance conferred by high level of bcl-2 alpha protein in human B lymphoblastoid cell. Oncogene. 1989;**4**(11):1331-1336

[32] Tsujimoto Y, Cossman J, Jaffe E, Croce CM. Involvement of the bcl-2 gene in human follicular lymphoma. Science. 1985;**228**(4706):1440-1443

[33] Tsujimoto Y, Finger LR, Yunis J, Nowell PC, Croce CM. Cloning of the chromosome breakpoint of neoplastic B cells with the t(14;18) chromosome translocation. Science. 1984;**226**(4678):1097-1099

[34] Warren CFA, Wong-Brown MW, Bowden NA. BCL-2 family isoforms in apoptosis and cancer. Cell Death & Disease. 2019;**10**(3):177

[35] Campbell KJ, Tait SWG. Targeting BCL-2 regulated apoptosis in cancer. Open Biology. 2018;**8**(5):180002

[36] Frenzel A, Grespi F, Chmelewskij W, Villunger A. Bcl2 family proteins in carcinogenesis and the treatment of cancer. Apoptosis. 2009;**14**(4):584-596

[37] Banerjee D. Genasense (Genta Inc). Current Opinion in Investigational Drugs. 2001;**2**(4):574-580

[38] O'Brien S, Moore JO, Boyd TE, Larratt LM, Skotnicki A, Koziner B, et al. Randomized phase III trial of fludarabine plus cyclophosphamide with or without oblimersen sodium (Bcl-2 antisense) in patients with relapsed or refractory chronic lymphocytic leukemia. Journal of Clinical Oncology. 2007;**25**(9):1114-1120

[39] Durig J, Duhrsen U, Klein-Hitpass L, Worm J, Hansen JB, Orum H, et al. The novel antisense Bcl-2 inhibitor SPC2996 causes rapid leukemic cell clearance and immune activation in chronic lymphocytic leukemia. Leukemia. 2011;**25**(4):638-647

[40] Green DR. A BH3 mimetic for killing cancer cells. Cell. 2016;**165**(7): 1560

[41] Pollyea DA, Amaya M, Strati P, Konopleva MY. Venetoclax for AML: Changing the treatment paradigm. Blood Advances. 2019;**3**(24):4326-4335

[42] Andrews DW, Judy KD, Scott CB, Garcia S, Harshyne LA, Kenyon L, et al. Phase Ib clinical trial of IGV-001 for patients with newly diagnosed glioblastoma. Clinical Cancer Research. 2021;**27**(7):1912-1922

[43] Young RM, Jamshidi A, Davis G, Sherman JH. Current trends in the surgical management and treatment of adult glioblastoma. Annals of Translational Medicine. 2015;**3**(9):121

[44] Stupp R, Hegi ME, Mason WP, van den Bent MJ, Taphoorn MJ, Janzer RC, et al. Effects of radiotherapy with concomitant and adjuvant temozolomide versus radiotherapy alone on survival in glioblastoma in a randomised phase III study: 5-year analysis of the EORTC-NCIC trial. The Lancet Oncology. 2009;**10**(5):459-466

[45] Larsson O, Girnita A, Girnita L. Role of insulin-like growth factor 1 receptor signalling in cancer. British Journal of Cancer. 2005;**92**(12):2097-2101

[46] Scartozzi M, Bianconi M, Maccaroni E, Giampieri R, Del Prete M, Berardi R, et al. State of the art and future perspectives for the use of insulin-like growth factor receptor 1 (IGF-1R) targeted treatment strategies in solid tumors. Discovery Medicine. 2011;**11**(57):144-153

[47] Philippou A, Armakolas A, Koutsilieris M. Evidence for the possible biological significance of the igf-1 gene alternative splicing in prostate cancer. Frontiers in Endocrinology (Lausanne). 2013;**4**:31

[48] Philippou A, Christopoulos PF, Koutsilieris DM. Clinical studies in humans targeting the various components of the IGF system show lack of efficacy in the treatment of cancer. Mutation Research, Reviews in Mutation Research. 2017;**772**:105-122

[49] Harshyne LA, Hooper KM, Andrews EG, Nasca BJ, Kenyon LC, Andrews DW, et al. Glioblastoma exosomes and IGF-1R/AS-ODN are immunogenic stimuli in a translational research immunotherapy paradigm. Cancer Immunology, Immunotherapy. 2015;**64**(3):299-309

[50] Morin-Brureau M, Hooper KM, Prosniak M, Sauma S, Harshyne LA, Andrews DW, et al. Enhancement of glioma-specific immunity in mice by "NOBEL", an insulin-like growth factor 1 receptor antisense oligodeoxynucleotide. Cancer Immunology, Immunotherapy. 2015;**64**(4):447-457

[51] Andrews DW, Resnicoff M, Flanders AE, Kenyon L, Curtis M, Merli G, et al. Results of a pilot study involving the use of an antisense oligodeoxynucleotide directed against the insulin-like growth factor type I receptor in malignant astrocytomas. Journal of Clinical Oncology. 2001;**19**(8):2189-2200

[52] Iaccarino C, Orlandi E, Ruggeri F, Nicoli D, Torricelli F, Maggi M, et al. Prognostic value of MGMT promoter status in non-resectable glioblastoma after adjuvant therapy. Clinical Neurology and Neurosurgery. 2015;**132**:1-8

[53] Hermisson M, Klumpp A, Wick W, Wischhusen J, Nagel G, Roos W, et al. O6-methylguanine DNA methyltransferase and p53 status predict temozolomide sensitivity in human malignant glioma cells. Journal of Neurochemistry. 2006;**96**(3):766-776

[54] Hegi ME, Diserens AC, Gorlia T, Hamou MF, de Tribolet N, Weller M, et al. MGMT gene silencing and benefit from temozolomide in glioblastoma. The New England Journal of Medicine. 2005;**352**(10):997-1003

[55] Tolcher AW, Papadopoulos KP, Patnaik A, Rasco DW, Martinez D, Wood DL, et al. Safety and activity of DCR-MYC, a first-in-class dicer-substrate small interfering RNA (DsiRNA) targeting MYC, in a phase I study in patients with advanced solid tumors. Journal of Clinical Oncology. 2015;**33**(15):Suppl11006

[56] Liu Z, Yoshimi A, Wang J, Cho H, Chun-Wei Lee S, Ki M, et al. Mutations in the RNA splicing factor SF3B1 promote tumorigenesis through MYC stabilization. Cancer Discovery. 2020;**10**(6):806-821

[57] Yoshimi A, Abdel-Wahab O. Molecular pathways: Understanding and targeting mutant spliceosomal proteins. Clinical Cancer Research. 2017;**23**(2):336-341

[58] Yoshimi A, Abdel-Wahab O. Splicing factor mutations in MDS RARS and MDS/MPN-RS-T. International Journal of Hematology. 2017;**105**(6):720-731

[59] Golan T, Khvalevsky EZ, Hubert A, Gabai RM, Hen N, Segal A, et al. RNAi therapy targeting KRAS in combination with chemotherapy for locally advanced pancreatic cancer patients. Oncotarget. 2015;**6**(27):24560-24570

[60] Varghese AM, Ang C, Dimaio CJ, Javle MM, Gutierrez M, Yarom N, et al. A phase II study of siG12D-LODER in combination with chemotherapy in patients with locally advanced pancreatic cancer (PROTACT). Journal of Clinical Oncology. 2020;**38**(15):SupplTPS4672

[61] Bonneau E, Neveu B, Kostantin E, Tsongalis GJ, De Guire V. How close are miRNAs from clinical practice? A perspective on the diagnostic and therapeutic market. EJIFCC. 2019;**30**(2):114-127

[62] Reid G, Pel ME, Kirschner MB, Cheng YY, Mugridge N, Weiss J, et al. Restoring expression of miR-16: A novel approach to therapy for malignant pleural mesothelioma. Annals of Oncology. 2013;**24**(12):3128-3135

[63] Kluiver J, Poppema S, de Jong D, Blokzijl T, Harms G, Jacobs S, et al. BIC and miR-155 are highly expressed in Hodgkin, primary mediastinal and diffuse large B cell lymphomas. The Journal of Pathology. 2005;**207**(2):243-249

[64] Eis PS, Tam W, Sun L, Chadburn A, Li Z, Gomez MF, et al. Accumulation of miR-155 and BIC RNA in human B cell lymphomas. Proceedings of the National Academy of Sciences of the United States of America. 2005;**102**(10):3627-3632

[65] Gerloff D, Grundler R, Wurm AA, Brauer-Hartmann D, Katzerke C, Hartmann JU, et al. NF-kappaB/STAT5/miR-155 network targets PU.1 in FLT3-ITD-driven acute myeloid leukemia. Leukemia. 2015;**29**(3):535-547

[66] Yamanaka Y, Tagawa H, Takahashi N, Watanabe A, Guo YM, Iwamoto K, et al. Aberrant overexpression of microRNAs activate AKT signaling via down-regulation of tumor suppressors in natural killer-cell lymphoma/leukemia. Blood. 2009;**114**(15):3265-3275

[67] Wang Y, Lee CG. MicroRNA and cancer—Focus on apoptosis. Journal of Cellular and Molecular Medicine. 2009;**13**(1):12-23

[68] Valeri N, Gasparini P, Fabbri M, Braconi C, Veronese A, Lovat F, et al. Modulation of mismatch repair and genomic stability by miR-155. Proceedings of the National Academy of Sciences of the United States of America. 2010;**107**(15):6982-6987

[69] Babar IA, Czochor J, Steinmetz A, Weidhaas JB, Glazer PM, Slack FJ. Inhibition of hypoxia-induced miR-155 radiosensitizes hypoxic lung cancer cells. Cancer Biology & Therapy. 2011;**12**(10):908-914

[70] Babar IA, Cheng CJ, Booth CJ, Liang X, Weidhaas JB, Saltzman WM, et al. Nanoparticle-based therapy in an in vivo microRNA-155 (miR-155)-dependent mouse model of lymphoma. Proceedings of the National Academy of Sciences of the United States of America. 2012;**109**(26):E1695-E1704

[71] O'Connell RM, Rao DS, Chaudhuri AA, Boldin MP, Taganov KD, Nicoll J, et al. Sustained expression of microRNA-155 in hematopoietic stem cells causes a myeloproliferative disorder. The Journal of Experimental Medicine. 2008;**205**(3):585-594

[72] Costinean S, Zanesi N, Pekarsky Y, Tili E, Volinia S, Heerema N, et al. Pre-B cell proliferation and lymphoblastic leukemia/high-grade lymphoma in E(mu)-miR155 transgenic mice.

Proceedings of the National Academy of Sciences of the United States of America. 2006;**103**(18):7024-7029

[73] O'Connell RM, Chaudhuri AA, Rao DS, Baltimore D. Inositol phosphatase SHIP1 is a primary target of miR-155. Proceedings of the National Academy of Sciences of the United States of America. 2009;**106**(17):7113-7118

[74] Yang Y, Yang L, Liang X, Zhu G. MicroRNA-155 promotes atherosclerosis inflammation via targeting SOCS1. Cellular Physiology and Biochemistry. 2015;**36**(4):1371-1381

[75] Huang X, Shen Y, Liu M, Bi C, Jiang C, Iqbal J, et al. Quantitative proteomics reveals that miR-155 regulates the PI3K-AKT pathway in diffuse large B-cell lymphoma. The American Journal of Pathology. 2012;**181**(1):26-33

[76] Ma X, Becker Buscaglia LE, Barker JR, Li Y. MicroRNAs in NF-kappaB signaling. Journal of Molecular Cell Biology. 2011;**3**(3):159-166

[77] Kopp KL, Ralfkiaer U, Gjerdrum LM, Helvad R, Pedersen IH, Litman T, et al. STAT5-mediated expression of oncogenic miR-155 in cutaneous T-cell lymphoma. Cell Cycle. 2013;**12**(12):1939-1947

[78] Seto AG, Beatty X, Lynch JM, Hermreck M, Tetzlaff M, Duvic M, et al. Cobomarsen, an oligonucleotide inhibitor of miR-155, co-ordinately regulates multiple survival pathways to reduce cellular proliferation and survival in cutaneous T-cell lymphoma. British Journal of Haematology. 2018;**183**(3):428-444

[79] Foss FM, Querfeld C, Porcu P, Kim YH, Pacheco T, Halwani AS, et al. Phase 1 trial evaluating MRG-106, a synthetic inhibitor of microRNA-155, in patients with cutaneous t-cell lymphoma (CTCL). Journal of Clinical Oncology. 2017;**35**(15):Suppl7564

[80] Bader AG. miR-34—A microRNA replacement therapy is headed to the clinic. Frontiers in Genetics. 2012;**3**:120

[81] Li H, Rokavec M, Jiang L, Horst D, Hermeking H. Antagonistic effects of p53 and HIF1A on microRNA-34a regulation of PPP1R11 and STAT3 and hypoxia-induced epithelial to mesenchymal transition in colorectal cancer cells. Gastroenterology. 2017;**153**(2):505-520

[82] Yang P, Li QJ, Feng Y, Zhang Y, Markowitz GJ, Ning S, et al. TGF-beta-miR-34a-CCL22 signaling-induced Treg cell recruitment promotes venous metastases of HBV-positive hepatocellular carcinoma. Cancer Cell. 2012;**22**(3):291-303

[83] Siemens H, Jackstadt R, Hunten S, Kaller M, Menssen A, Gotz U, et al. miR-34 and SNAIL form a double-negative feedback loop to regulate epithelial-mesenchymal transitions. Cell Cycle. 2011;**10**(24):4256-4271

[84] Li Y, Guessous F, Zhang Y, Dipierro C, Kefas B, Johnson E, et al. MicroRNA-34a inhibits glioblastoma growth by targeting multiple oncogenes. Cancer Research. 2009;**69**(19):7569-7576

[85] Guessous F, Zhang Y, Kofman A, Catania A, Li Y, Schiff D, et al. microRNA-34a is tumor suppressive in brain tumors and glioma stem cells. Cell Cycle. 2010;**9**(6):1031-1036

[86] Bu P, Chen KY, Chen JH, Wang L, Walters J, Shin YJ, et al. A microRNA miR-34a-regulated bimodal switch targets notch in colon cancer stem cells. Cell Stem Cell. 2013;**12**(5):602-615

[87] Beg MS, Brenner AJ, Sachdev J, Borad M, Kang YK, Stoudemire J, et al. Phase I study of MRX34, a liposomal

miR-34a mimic, administered twice weekly in patients with advanced solid tumors. Investigational New Drugs. 2017;**35**(2):180-188

[88] Ghia P, Strola G, Granziero L, Geuna M, Guida G, Sallusto F, et al. Chronic lymphocytic leukemia B cells are endowed with the capacity to attract CD4+, CD40L+ T cells by producing CCL22. European Journal of Immunology. 2002;**32**(5):1403-1413

[89] Nishio M, Endo T, Tsukada N, Ohata J, Kitada S, Reed JC, et al. Nurselike cells express BAFF and APRIL, which can promote survival of chronic lymphocytic leukemia cells via a paracrine pathway distinct from that of SDF-1alpha. Blood. 2005;**106**(3):1012-1020

[90] Burger JA, Tsukada N, Burger M, Zvaifler NJ, Dell'Aquila M, Kipps TJ. Blood-derived nurse-like cells protect chronic lymphocytic leukemia B cells from spontaneous apoptosis through stromal cell-derived factor-1. Blood. 2000;**96**(8):2655-2663

[91] Burger JA, Burger M, Kipps TJ. Chronic lymphocytic leukemia B cells express functional CXCR4 chemokine receptors that mediate spontaneous migration beneath bone marrow stromal cells. Blood. 1999;**94**(11):3658-3667

[92] Kurtova AV, Balakrishnan K, Chen R, Ding W, Schnabl S, Quiroga MP, et al. Diverse marrow stromal cells protect CLL cells from spontaneous and drug-induced apoptosis: Development of a reliable and reproducible system to assess stromal cell adhesion-mediated drug resistance. Blood. 2009;**114**(20):4441-4450

[93] Lagneaux L, Delforge A, Bron D, De Bruyn C, Stryckmans P. Chronic lymphocytic leukemic B cells but not normal B cells are rescued from apoptosis by contact with normal bone marrow stromal cells. Blood. 1998;**91**(7):2387-2396

[94] Nagasawa T, Kikutani H, Kishimoto T. Molecular cloning and structure of a pre-B-cell growth-stimulating factor. Proceedings of the National Academy of Sciences of the United States of America. 1994;**91**(6):2305-2309

[95] O'Hayre M, Salanga CL, Kipps TJ, Messmer D, Dorrestein PC, Handel TM. Elucidating the CXCL12/CXCR4 signaling network in chronic lymphocytic leukemia through phosphoproteomics analysis. PLoS One. 2010;**5**(7):e11716

[96] Burger M, Hartmann T, Krome M, Rawluk J, Tamamura H, Fujii N, et al. Small peptide inhibitors of the CXCR4 chemokine receptor (CD184) antagonize the activation, migration, and antiapoptotic responses of CXCL12 in chronic lymphocytic leukemia B cells. Blood. 2005;**106**(5):1824-1830

[97] Andritsos LA, Byrd JC, Cheverton P, Wu J, Sivina M, Kipps TJ, et al. A multicenter phase 1 study of plerixafor and rituximab in patients with chronic lymphocytic leukemia. Leukemia & Lymphoma. 2019;**60**(14):3461-3469

[98] Eulberg D, Klussmann S. Spiegelmers: Biostable aptamers. Chembiochem. 2003;**4**(10):979-983

[99] Klussmann S, Nolte A, Bald R, Erdmann VA, Furste JP. Mirror-image RNA that binds D-adenosine. Nature Biotechnology. 1996;**14**(9):1112-1115

[100] Steurer M, Montillo M, Scarfo L, Mauro FR, Andel J, Wildner S, et al. Olaptesed pegol (NOX-A12) with bendamustine and rituximab: A phase IIa study in patients with relapsed/refractory

chronic lymphocytic leukemia. Haematologica. 2019;**104**(10):2053-2060

[101] Jain N, Balakrishnan K, Ferrajoli A, O'Brien SM, Burger JA, Kadia TM, et al. A phase I-II trial of fludarabine, bendamustine and rituximab (FBR) in previously treated patients with CLL. Oncotarget. 2017;**8**(13):22104-22112

[102] Visco C, Finotto S, Pomponi F, Sartori R, Laveder F, Trentin L, et al. The combination of rituximab, bendamustine, and cytarabine for heavily pretreated relapsed/refractory cytogenetically high-risk patients with chronic lymphocytic leukemia. American Journal of Hematology. 2013;**88**(4):289-293

[103] Ludwig H, Weisel K, Petrucci MT, Leleu X, Cafro AM, Garderet L, et al. Olaptesed pegol, an anti-CXCL12/SDF-1 Spiegelmer, alone and with bortezomib-dexamethasone in relapsed/refractory multiple myeloma: A phase IIa study. Leukemia. 2017;**31**(4):997-1000

[104] Roccaro AM, Sacco A, Purschke WG, Moschetta M, Buchner K, Maasch C, et al. SDF-1 inhibition targets the bone marrow niche for cancer therapy. Cell Reports. 2014;**9**(1):118-128

[105] Bouyssou JM, Ghobrial IM, Roccaro AM. Targeting SDF-1 in multiple myeloma tumor microenvironment. Cancer Letters. 2016;**380**(1):315-318

[106] Palumbo A, Chanan-Khan A, Weisel K, Nooka AK, Masszi T, Beksac M, et al. Daratumumab, bortezomib, and dexamethasone for multiple myeloma. The New England Journal of Medicine. 2016;**375**(8):754-766

[107] Dimopoulos MA, Moreau P, Palumbo A, Joshua D, Pour L, Hajek R, et al. Carfilzomib and dexamethasone versus bortezomib and dexamethasone for patients with relapsed or refractory multiple myeloma (ENDEAVOR): A randomised, phase 3, open-label, multicentre study. The Lancet Oncology. 2016;**17**(1):27-38

[108] San-Miguel JF, Hungria VT, Yoon SS, Beksac M, Dimopoulos MA, Elghandour A, et al. Panobinostat plus bortezomib and dexamethasone versus placebo plus bortezomib and dexamethasone in patients with relapsed or relapsed and refractory multiple myeloma: A multicentre, randomised, double-blind phase 3 trial. The Lancet Oncology. 2014;**15**(11):1195-1206

[109] Harrison SJ, Quach H, Link E, Feng HB, Dean J, Copeman M, et al. The addition of dexamethasone to bortezomib for patients with relapsed multiple myeloma improves outcome but ongoing maintenance therapy has minimal benefit. American Journal of Hematology. 2015;**90**(5):E86-E91

[110] Arnulf B, Pylypenko H, Grosicki S, Karamanesht I, Leleu X, van de Velde H, et al. Updated survival analysis of a randomized phase III study of subcutaneous versus intravenous bortezomib in patients with relapsed multiple myeloma. Haematologica. 2012;**97**(12):1925-1928

[111] Richardson PG, Sonneveld P, Schuster M, Irwin D, Stadtmauer E, Facon T, et al. Extended follow-up of a phase 3 trial in relapsed multiple myeloma: Final time-to-event results of the APEX trial. Blood. 2007;**110**(10):3557-3560

[112] Ghobrial IM, Shain KH, Laubach J, Henrick P, Vredenburg J, Crilley P, et al. Final results of the phase I/II study of chemosensitization using the CXCR4 inhibitor plerixafor in combination with bortezomib in patients with relapsed or relapsed/refractory multiple myeloma. Blood. 2015;**126**(23):4256

[113] Ghobrial IM, Perez R, Baz R, Richardson PG, Anderson KC, Sabbatini P, et al. Phase Ib study of the novel anti-CXCR4 antibody ulocuplumab (BMS-936564) in combination with lenalidomide plus low-dose dexamethasone, or with bortezomib plus dexamethasone in subjects with relapsed or refractory multiple myeloma. Blood. 2014;**124**(21):3483

[114] Rhym LH, Anderson DG. Nanoscale delivery platforms for RNA therapeutics: Challenges and the current state of the art. Med (N Y). 2022;**3**(3):167-187

Section 4

RNA Drugs for Rare Diseases

Chapter 6

RNA Interference Applications for Machado-Joseph Disease

José M. Codêsso, Carlos A. Matos and Clévio Nóbrega

Abstract

Machado-Joseph disease (MJD), also named spinocerebellar ataxia type 3 (SCA3), is a dominantly inherited neurodegenerative disease caused by abnormal CAG expansions in *MJD1* gene, which translate to an overexpanded tract of glutamines in the ataxin-3 (ATXN3) protein. Since the identification of the causative gene, a huge effort was made toward the development of animal models for MJD/SCA3, to increase the understanding of the molecular mechanisms underpinning disease pathogenesis, and to develop therapeutic strategies for the disease. Nevertheless, until now there are no therapies available capable of stopping or delaying the disease progression, which culminates with the death of the patients. Therefore, there is an urgent unmet need for therapeutic solutions, for which gene therapy stands out. The RNA interference (RNAi) mechanism discovery allowed the identification of small RNA molecules with the ability to regulate gene expression. For gene therapy, RNAi provided a way to silence mutant genes, which are particularly useful in dominantly inherited diseases. In the last years, several studies have focused on using RNAi molecules to target mutant ATXN3. The results showed that this could be an efficient and safe strategy for modifying MJD/SCA3 progression. Now, an additional effort must be done to translate these results into clinical trials.

Keywords: Machado-Joseph disease/spinocerebellar ataxia type 3, ataxin-3, RNA interference technology, (non-) allele-specific gene silencing, exogenous small interfering RNAs, short hairpin RNAs, artificial microRNAs, microRNA mimics

1. Introduction

1.1 Machado-Joseph disease

Machado-Joseph disease (MJD), also named spinocerebellar ataxia type 3 (SCA3), is an inherited and rare neurodegenerative disease, usually with adult-onset, and is considered the most common autosomal dominant ataxia worldwide. It is part of the group of polyglutamine (polyQ) disorders. The group currently includes nine disorders — Huntington's disease (HD), dentatorubral pallidoluysian atrophy (DRPLA), spinal and bulbar muscular atrophy (SBMA), and six different spinocerebellar ataxias (SCA1/2/3/6/7/17). These disorders are caused by abnormal expansions of the CAG trinucleotide in the coding region of the causative genes, which are translated into abnormally long polyQ tracts in the respective proteins [1–4]. MJD/SCA3 was

IntechOpen

initially described in Portuguese descendants in the United States. Among SCAs, its relative frequency is higher in countries such as Brazil [5], Portugal [6, 7], China [8], Germany [9], and Japan [10, 11]. In the Azores islands, the disease has the highest prevalence registered worldwide (1:140 on the small island of Flores) [12].

The main clinical manifestation of MJD/SCA3 is progressive cerebellar ataxia – motor incoordination that can affect balance, gait, and speech [13]. Other symptoms of the disease include a pyramidal syndrome with brisk deep tendon reflexes and spasticity; peripheral neuropathy with amyotrophy; oculomotor abnormalities with nystagmus, eyelid retraction and progressive external ophthalmoplegia; facial and lingual fasciculation; and extrapyramidal signs like dystonia and rigidity [14–18]. The neurodegenerative process in MJD/SCA3 affects multiple neuronal systems, particularly cerebellum, brainstem, basal ganglia, spinal cord, and some cranial nerves [19, 20].

MJD/SCA3 is caused by the abnormal expansion of the CAG trinucleotide in the coding region of the *MJD1* gene located on chromosome 14q32.1 [21]. The number of repeats is about 10–51 in healthy individuals and 55–87 in MJD/SCA3 patients, and there is a positive correlation between the CAG repeat number and both the severity and precocity of the symptoms, a neuropathological feature common to other polyQ disorders [22–24]. The MJD1 gene encodes ataxin-3 (ATXN3), a protein whose biochemical function seems to be associated with the UPS [25, 26]. Some studies also suggest that ATXN3 is involved in the regulation of transcription and in DNA repair mechanisms [27–30]. Upon translation, the mutation results in an abnormally long polyQ tract at the carboxylic terminus of ATXN3. The mutant protein then acquires toxic properties and initiates a cascade of molecular mechanisms that culminate in neurodegeneration. An important neuropathological hallmark of MJD/SCA3 is the accumulation of neuronal insoluble aggregates containing the mutant ATXN3, predominantly in the nucleus, both inside and outside of the areas affected by neurodegeneration. That is a key feature of all polyQ diseases [31–33].

There is no cure for MJD/SCA3. However, several therapeutic strategies (**Figure 1**) have been developed to counteract the disease pathogenesis at different stages, namely RNA interference (RNAi)-based approaches. Considering the pathological features, the strategies involve targeting (i) mutant mRNA, (ii) mutant protein aggregation, (iii) toxic proteolytic cleavage of mutant protein, (iv) protein clearance pathways (autophagy and ubiquitin-proteasome system), (v) posttranslational modifications, (vi) transcriptional dysregulation, (vii) mitochondrial dysfunction, (viii) calcium homeostasis, and (ix) neuroprotective pathways. In quite general terms, the RNAi technology constitutes a powerful tool that allows targeting the mutant ATXN3 mRNA, thereby controlling the mutant ATXN3 protein expression [34].

1.2 RNA interference mechanism

All scientific discoveries have precedents, and the RNAi mechanism was no exception. In the late 1980s and early 1990s, plant biologists, trying to genetically increase the purple pigmentation of petunias' flowers, were surprised when they noticed, not as expected, that introducing multiple extra copies of a gene that codes for "purple flowers," via *Agrobacterium*, led to plants with white or variegated flowers. Somehow, the introduced extra copies of the gene had silenced both themselves and the plants' own "purple-flower" gene [35, 36]. An explanation for these observations remained elusive until 1998 when Fire, Mello, and colleagues discovered the RNAi mechanism. The authors reported a selective and efficient silencing of a target gene using an exogenous and naked double-stranded RNA (dsRNA), in a sequence-specific manner, in

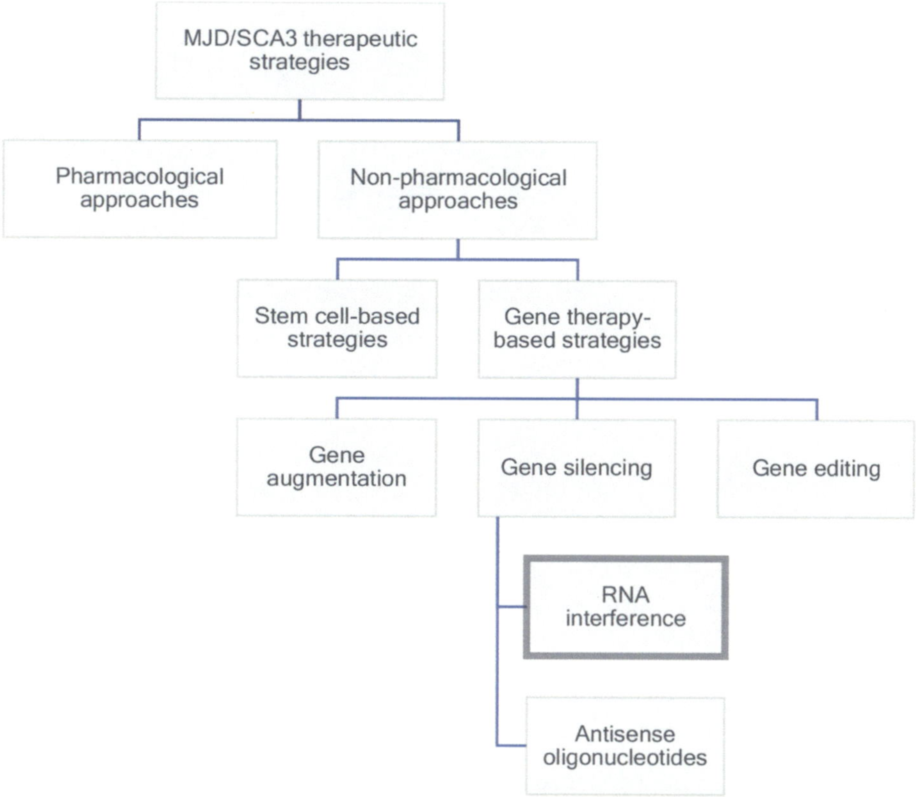

Figure 1.
Schematic representation of possible MJD/SCA3 therapeutic strategies, especially detailing the non-pharmacological approaches [34].

Caenorhabditis elegans. Additionally, they also observed that the dsRNA was substantially more effective at silencing the gene than was the corresponding single-stranded (ssRNA) antisense strand individually [37]. Regarding the petunias' experiments, the multiple copies of the gene introduced in the plant genome led to the generation of a homologous dsRNA, which, subsequently, mediated the silencing of both introduced and endogenous genes [38, 39].

Since then, the discovery of the RNAi mechanism, numerous studies have furthered our understanding of the RNAi mechanism, and how RNAi could be an extremely useful experimental tool for learning what genes do and for the development of potential therapeutic strategies.

1.2.1 Endogenous RNA interference mechanism

The endogenous RNAi mechanism is an evolutionarily conserved process used by cells to regulate gene expression. In general terms, the naturally occurring key molecules of the endogenous RNAi mechanism are categorized into three classes: microRNAs (miRNAs), endogenous small interfering RNAs (endo-siRNAs), and PIWI-interacting RNAs (piRNAs). The most extensively studied class is the class of the miRNAs. All those regulatory RNAs are small noncoding RNAs that have a particular homology for specific genes, and a wide variety of expression patterns, especially in a time and a cell or tissue-dependent manner [40–42].

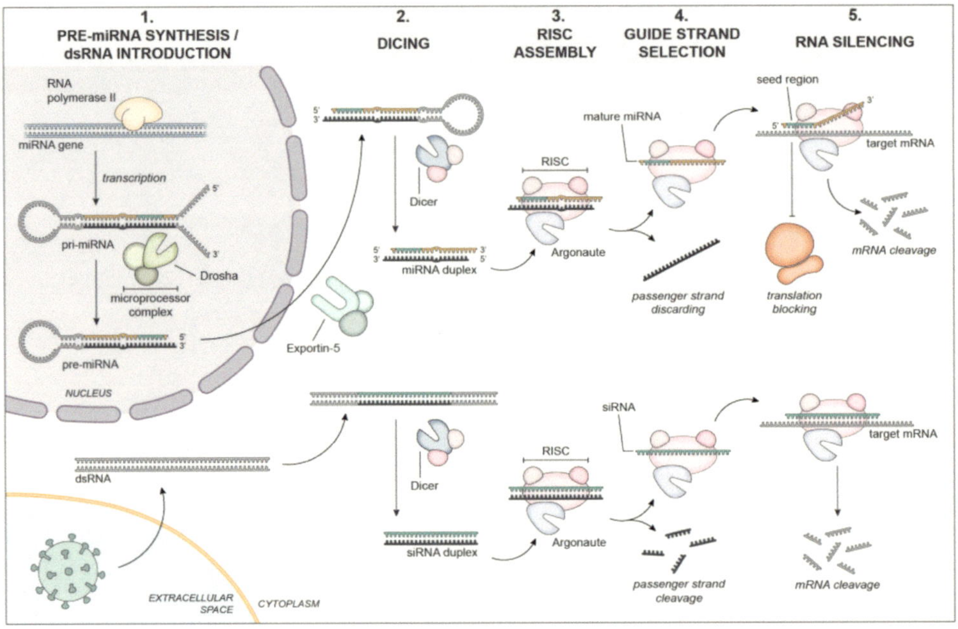

Figure 2.
Overview of the RNAi pathway depicting the two principal sub-pathways: the miRNA pathway and the siRNA pathway.

The endogenous RNAi mechanism (**Figure 2**) has been deeply implicated in several aspects of animal and plant development and their regular physiological functioning, namely cell differentiation, cell proliferation, and cell death. It has been involved in the pathophysiological processes of numerous diseases, as well. Additionally, the endogenous RNAi mechanism also provides antiviral "molecular defense" response and restricts "genomic parasites," such as transposable elements. It is known that RNAi can effectively protect hosts against viruses, by intercepting and inhibiting viral transcripts through miRNAs. RNAi can also protect cells against transposable elements, both by degrading the transcripts of transposable elements and by preventing the expression of transposable elements through heterochromatin formation [43–46].

In animals, the miRNA pathway, the most notorious pathway, can be divided into multiple steps. Initially, in the nucleus, the miRNA genes are transcribed into long primary transcripts, the primary miRNAs (pri-miRNAs), that have a stem-loop structure flanked by single-stranded regions corresponding to the 5′ end (with 7-methylguanosine) and 3′ end (with the poly-A tail). The transcription is generally processed by RNA polymerase II [47, 48]. Then, the pri-miRNAs are cleaved at the opposite extremity of the loop by Drosha, a ribonuclease type III (RNase III), generating miRNA precursors, the precursor miRNAs (pre-miRNAs), which maintain the stem-loop structure but with a 2-nucleotide 3′ overhang. During the process, Drosha forms an enzymatic complex with another protein, the dsRNA-binding protein DiGeorge syndrome critical region gene 8 (DGCR8), that stabilizes the pri-miRNAs. The complex mentioned above is known as a microprocessor [49–52]. Additional proteins, such as the enhancer of the rudimentary homolog (ERH), can also interact with the microprocessor, modulating its catalytic activity [53].

Still in the nucleus, the pre-miRNAs associate with the dsRNA-binding protein exportin-5 that transfers them to the cytoplasm, in the presence of the Ras-related nuclear- GTP-binding protein (Ran-GTP) [54, 55]. After the hydrolysis of GTP, the pre-miRNAs are released and intercepted by a cluster of proteins containing the RNase III Dicer and the dsRNA-binding proteins HIV-1 transactivating response (TAR)- RNA-binding protein (TRBP) and protein kinase R (PKR) activator (PACT). Dicer recognizes the 2-nucleotide 3′ overhang of the pre-miRNAs (through its Piwi-Argonaut-Zwille (PAZ) domain, an RNA-binding domain) and cleaves the loop extremity. That originates miRNAs duplexes of approximately 21–23 nucleotides in length (on each strand) harboring 2-nucleotide 3′ overhangs at both extremities. The proteins TRBP and PACT stabilize the pre-miRNAs during the process [56–59].

After the previous processing step catalyzed by Dicer, the cluster of proteins containing Dicer, TRBP, and PACT provides a structural landing platform for the recruitment of another protein, argonaute (habitually argonaute-2), which associates with the miRNA duplexes, recognizing the 2-nucleotide 3′ overhangs (like Dicer, argonaute has a PAZ domain). Altogether, the proteins above are the major members of the RNA-induced silencing complex (RISC), which mediates later the messenger RNA (mRNA) silencing. The RISC becomes active when only one of the strands of the miRNA duplexes (guide strand, antisense strand, mature miRNA, or simply miRNA or miR) remains associated with argonaute. The other strand (the passenger strand, the sense strand) is removed and rapidly degraded [60–62]. If the nucleotide-pairing between the two strands of the miRNA duplexes is imperfect, it seems to be argonaute itself, through its endonucleolytic strand-dissociating activity, which dissociates the guide strand and the passenger strand (the most likely pathway since the miRNA duplexes frequently have mismatches). If the nucleotide-pairing is perfect or near-perfect, it is suggested that RNA helicases, through their strand-unwinding activity, separate the two strands [63–65]. Experimental evidence suggests that miRNA duplexes dissociation starts at the extremity with the lowest thermodynamic stability. The strand that has its 5′ end at this extremity is the one that preferentially remains associated with argonaute, and acts later as a guide strand in the mRNA silencing [66].

The final step of the miRNA pathway occurs when the miRNAs bound to argonaute selectively recognize and bind to the target mRNAs, and then the miRNAs-mRNAs macrostructures are degraded. The specificity of the mRNA recognition derives primarily from the high-level complementarity of the nucleotide sequence comprising the nucleotides 2–8 of the 5′ end of the miRNAs, known as seed region, with the 3′ untranslated region (UTR) of the mRNAs (in general, but the miRNAs can also target coding regions). Moreover, some experimental data revealed an additional nucleotide sequence in the miRNAs, termed supplementary region, comprising at least the 13–16 nucleotides, that seems to be equally important in the specificity of the mRNA recognition, given the high-level complementarity with the 3′ UTR of the mRNAs, as well. The importance increases when the complementarity of the seed region is suboptimal. As a rule, except for the localized nucleotide sequences mentioned above, the complementarity of the remaining nucleotides of the miRNAs with the 3' UTR of the mRNAs is partial, and the occurrence of mismatches and bulges is common and naturally tolerated [67–70]. After the miRNAs selectively recognize and bind to the target mRNAs, the miRNAs-mRNAs macrostructures, along with argonaute, are transported to cytoplasmic compartments called processing bodies (P-bodies) that promote its degradation. In this way, the miRNAs lead to the silencing of the target mRNAs, inhibiting the translation (or, in fact, leading to the silencing of the corresponding genes) [71, 72].

Considering the endo-siRNA pathway, in animals, there are several dsRNAs sources, which constitute endo-siRNAs precursors and ultimately originate endo-siRNAs. These sources include i) pairs of transposable element transcripts, which are formed by two transcripts from a single transposable element bi-directionally transcribed [73, 74]; ii) pairs of cis-natural antisense transcripts (cis-NATs), which are formed by two overlapping transcripts from the same genomic locus) [75]; iii) pairs of trans-NATs (also known as gene-pseudogene pairs), which are formed by two overlapping transcripts from distinct genomic loci, usually a gene mRNA and a pseudogene transcript [76]; and iv) hairpin RNA transcripts with stem-loop structure, which result from the transcription of long inverted repeats [77]. The endo-siRNAs precursors are long dsRNAs and, once in the cytoplasm, they are processed by Dicer into smaller endo-siRNAs duplexes of around 20–23 nucleotides in length (on each strand). After the RISC assembly and the subsequent strand selection, the endo-siRNAs bound to argonaute selectively recognize and bind to the target RNAs, such as transposon transcripts or endogenous mRNAs. Then, the endo-siRNAs-RNAs macro-structures are directly cleaved by argonaute in the RISC. This differs from the miRNA pathway due to the high-level complementarity of the entire nucleotide sequence of the endo-siRNAs with the target RNAs [78–81].

The piRNA pathway was originally described in the *Drosophila* germline, and it has several features that distinguish it from miRNA and endo-siRNA pathways. First, in *Drosophila*, specific genomic loci, such as piRNA clusters, are transcribed into long antisense single-stranded piRNA precursors. After being transported to the cytoplasm, the endonuclease Zucchini (Zuc) (or mitochondrial phospholipase D6-MitoPLD — in mice and humans) processes the piRNA precursors into mature antisense piRNAs of approximately 25–33 nucleotides in length [82–85]. Then, the antisense piRNAs are loaded into PIWI proteins, a subgroup of argonaute proteins, and depending on the PIWI protein involved, the piRNAs have different fates. piRNAs bound to aubergine (Miwi in mice and Hiwi in humans) participate in a posttranscriptional gene silencing of target RNAs in the cytoplasm, such as transposon transcripts. In contrast, piRNAs bound to PIWI (Miwi2 in mice and Hiwi2 in humans) translocate to the nucleus and, there, promote transcriptional gene silencing. As a rule, the posttranscriptional gene silencing mediated by piRNAs is a slicer-dependent mechanism that depends on catalytically active aubergine. By contrast, the transcriptional gene silencing mediated by piRNAs does not involve the cleavage of the target. Instead, it leads to a target shutdown through chromatin modifications, such as repressive histone marks and DNA methylation [82, 83, 86–89].

During posttranscriptional gene silencing, additional antisense piRNAs are generated through an amplification mechanism termed the ping-pong cycle. In the cytoplasm, aubergine, through its normal slicer activity, naturally generate transposon transcript fragments that are used in the ping-pong cycle as sense piRNAs intermediates. Following a maturation process, which includes trimming to the appropriate length, the sense piRNAs intermediates originate mature sense piRNAs. Then, the sense piRNAs are loaded into the PIWI protein argonaute-3 (Mili in mice and Hili in humans) that subsequently cleaves the piRNA precursors, producing more antisense piRNAs with sequences identical, or near-identical to the original triggers. The ping-pong cycle continues with the aubergine loading once again [82, 83, 90–92].

1.2.2 RNA interference mechanism mediated by artificial RNA effector molecules

The endogenous RNAi mechanism can be artificially triggered to induce specific gene silencing by different RNA effector molecules: exogenous (exo)-siRNAs, short hairpin RNAs (shRNAs), artificial miRNAs, and miRNA mimics [93]. The exo-siRNAs are usually double-stranded molecules of around 21–23 nucleotides in length, chemically synthesized, and their guide strand has full complementarity with the target mRNAs. The delivery occurs using non-expression-based systems, including nanoparticles, such as lipid-based nanoparticles or polymer-derived nanoparticles. The exo-siRNAs are designed to mimic miRNA duplexes and enter the endogenous RNAi mechanism upon being loaded into the RISC in the cytoplasm. Following the strand selection, the passenger strand is degraded, whereas the guide strand bound to argonaute associates with specific complementary mRNAs, targeting them for direct cleavage by argonaute [94, 95]. The exo-siRNAs can be incorporated into stem-loop structures and originate shRNAs, when integrated into an artificial stem-loop, mimicking pre-miRNAs, or artificial miRNAs, when integrated into a backbone that derives from a natural pri-miRNA backbone, mimicking a pri-miRNA. Like exo-siRNAs, the guide strand of shRNAs and artificial miRNAs typically has full complementarity with the target mRNAs. Both molecules are delivered by expression-based systems, such as plasmids or viral vectors. Following viral-mediated transduction and subsequent transcription within the nucleus, the shRNAs are translocated to the cytoplasm by exportin-5. Then occurs Dicer processing and incorporation into the RISC. The next steps are like those of exo-siRNAs. In turn, the artificial miRNA genesis is most upstream and requires an additional step — Drosha processing within the nucleus [96, 97]. The miRNA mimics are synthetic double-stranded molecules comprising a guide strand that is designed to recognize and bind to a target mRNA with partial complementarity, as a mature miRNA. In fact, the guide strand typically corresponds to a naturally occurring mature miRNA, for a proper miRNA replacement and a natural mode of action silencing target mRNAs. The miRNAs mimics can be directly delivered by non-expression-based vectors or delivered by expression-based vectors. Depending on the delivery method, the miRNA mimics enter the endogenous RNAi mechanism as mentioned for the previous effector molecules [98, 99].

A possible categorization of the delivery systems is to divide them into expression-based vectors and non-expression-based vectors. The expression-based vectors are considered much more efficient, especially the viral vectors, by allowing the effector molecules to permanently silence a target gene upon one single administration. In contrast, the non-expression-based vectors are generally safer and easier to produce. Their transient nature allows an interruption of the administration [100].

Although RNAi technology has a widely recognized potential as a therapeutic strategy, its efficiency has been questioned due to unintended effects that culminate in cell dysfunction or even animal death [101]. The cytotoxic effects include i) the saturation of the endogenous RNAi processing machinery, which derives from the overexpression of the effector molecules [101, 102]; ii) the induction of the immune response, due to the activation of cellular sensors that typically recognize foreign RNA and DNA, which then leads to the production of proinflammatory cytokines and interferons [103, 104]; and iii) potential off-target effects, which in general derive from unintended interactions between the guide strand of the effector molecules and other transcripts containing complementary sequences [105, 106].

2. Therapeutic strategies for Machado-Joseph disease based on RNA interference

MJD/SCA3 is caused by a specific genetic mutation — a CAG repeat expansion — in the coding region of the *MJD1* gene, similar to other polyQ disorders on their causative genes, which trigger various pathogenic mechanisms. Due to their dominant monogenic nature, RNAi technology provides a great opportunity to inhibit the mutant gene expression, at the earliest steps, over the mRNA, which could prevent the disease onset or progression. RNAi technology establishes not only a way to inhibit the toxic effects of the mutant protein, but also a way to inhibit the probable toxic effects of the mutant RNA [107]. Indeed, RNA toxicity has emerged as a crucial factor in the pathogenesis of polyQ disorders [108]. In MJD/SCA3, some studies have reported a mutant ATXN3 RNA-derived toxicity in *Drosophila*, *Caenorhabditis elegans,* and different mouse models [109–111].

Considering all this, several therapeutic strategies for MJD/SCA3 based on RNAi have been conceived, involving gene silencing mediated by exo-siRNAs and shRNAs (**Table 1**) and gene silencing mediated by artificial miRNAs and miRNA mimics (**Table 2**).

2.1 Exogenous small interfering RNA and short hairpin RNA-mediated gene silencing

The gene silencing mediated by exo-siRNAs and shRNAs, applied to MJD/SCA3, can be divided into two distinct categories: (i) non-allele-specific gene silencing and (ii) allele-specific gene silencing. The non-allele-specific silencing constitutes the most straightforward methodology, and unselectively silences both wild-type and mutant genes. On the other hand, allele-specific silencing is a more accurate methodology that allows the selective silencing of the mutant gene. The allele distinction is particularly important when the wild-type protein is essential for cellular function. To accomplish the allele distinction, differences between both transcripts of the genes, such as single-nucleotide polymorphisms (SNPs) and the CAG repeat itself, are used to design the effector molecules [128, 129].

2.1.1 Non-allele-specific gene silencing

In a non-allele-specific gene silencing approach on MJD/SCA3, following *in vitro* validation of its efficacy, a shRNA designed to target both human wild-type and mutant ATXN3 proved to be safe and efficient in a lentiviral rat model. This lentiviral model was generated through the stereotaxic injection of lentivirus encoding the human mutant ATXN3 in the striatum of wild-type animals. The administration of the shRNA encoded by lentivirus led to a reduction of the human mutant ATXN3 levels and to a significant decrease of the neuropathological inclusions [112].

In another study, an exo-siRNA targeting the CAG repeat expansion and delivered by a liposome-based vector strongly reduced both mutant ATXN3 and wild-type ATXN3 protein levels, in MJD/SCA3 patient-derived fibroblasts. Furthermore, similar results were obtained for huntingtin, in a HD context, with the same exo-siRNA. It shows that a gene silencing approach targeting the CAG repeat expansion can be beneficial for different polyQ diseases [113].

Mouse and *Caenorhabditis elegans* knockout models for ATXN3, created to evaluate the physiological functions of this protein, showed to be viable and to have no major abnormalities [130, 131]. Nevertheless, a cellular experiment with a similar intent revealed that the absence of ATXN3 impacts the expression of a large set of genes involved in multiple signaling transduction pathways, and that may result in detrimental consequences [132]. Altogether, the experimental data above suggest that the optimal and safest gene silencing approach for MJD/SCA3 may be an allele-specific silencing of the mutant ATXN3, whenever possible, maintaining the endogenous ATXN3 functional.

Effector molecule	Allele specificity	Expression system	Delivery system	Reference
shRNA	Non-allele-specific	HEK 293T[1] cell model and lentiviral mouse model	Transfection and lentivirus-mediated transduction	[112]
exo-siRNA targeting CAG repeat expansion	Non-allele-specific	Patient-derived fibroblasts	Transfection	[113]
exo-siRNAs and shRNAs targeting G/C SNP	Allele-specific	COS-7[2] cell model	Transfection and adenovirus-mediated transduction	[114]
exo-siRNA targeting G/C SNP	Allele-specific	HEK 293T cell model	Transfection	[115]
shRNA targeting G/C SNP	Allele-specific	HEK 293T cell model, lentiviral rat and mouse models, and transgenic mouse model	Transfection and lentivirus-mediated transduction	[116–118]
exo-siRNA targeting G/C SNP	Allele-specific	Neuro2a cell model, lentiviral and transgenic mouse models	SNALP-mediated transfection	[119]
exo-siRNAs targeting CAG repeat expansion	Allele-specific	Patient-derived fibroblasts	Transfection	[120]
shRNA targeting CAG repeat expansion	Allele-specific	Patient-derived fibroblasts	Lentivirus-mediated transduction	[121]
ss-exo-siRNAs targeting CAG repeat expansion	Allele-specific	Patient-derived fibroblasts	Transfection	[122]

[1]*Human embryonic kidney 293T (HEK293T)*
[2]*CV-1 simian cells transformed by an origin-defective mutant of SV40 (COS-7)*

Table 1.
exo-siRNA and shRNA-mediated gene silencing approaches for MJD/SCA3.

Effector molecule	Allele specificity	Expression system	Delivery system	Reference
Artificial miRNA targeting 3′ UTR of ATXN3	Non-allele-specific	Transgenic mouse model	AAV-mediated transduction	[123, 124]
Artificial miRNAs targeting exons within ATXN3	Non-allele-specific	Heterozygous knock-in mouse model	AAV-mediated transduction	[125]
miR-25 mimic	(Naturally) non-specific	HEK 293T[1] cell model	Transfection	[126]
mir-9, mir-181a and mir-494 mimics	(Naturally) non-specific	HEK 293T cell model and lentiviral mouse model	Transfection and lentivirus-mediated transduction	[127]

[1]*Human embryonic kidney 293T (HEK293T)*

Table 2.
Artificial miRNA and miRNA mimic-mediated gene silencing approaches for MJD/SCA3.

2.1.2 Allele-specific gene silencing

Extensive efforts on MJD/SCA3 have been made toward allele-specific silencing of the mutant ATXN3. Several allele-specific approaches have been focused on a SNP (**G987**GG → **C987**GG) located at the 3′ end of the gene, in linkage disequilibrium and immediately following the CAG repeat expansion. The wild-type ATXN3 gene has a **G** at position 987, whereas the mutant ATXN3 gene has a **C** at that position. All the remaining sequence is identical in both genes. The **G/C** SNP is present in approximately 70% of MJD/SCA3 patients [133–135]. Taking into consideration the **G/C** SNP, Miller and colleagues designed exo-siRNAs and shRNAs encoded by plasmids or adenovirus, and then accomplished an allele-specific silencing of the mutant ATXN3 in cell cultures, with the three experimental systems. The mutant ATXN3 levels were effectively reduced, the accumulation of aggregated protein decreased and only slight effects on the wild-type ATXN3 levels were detected [114]. Similarly, Li and colleagues also created an exo-siRNA targeting the **G/C** SNP that led to a reduction of the mutant ATXN3 levels, with minimal impact on the wild-type ATXN3 levels, in a cellular model [115].

Later it was demonstrated in rodent models of MJD/SCA3 that it is possible to selectively and efficiently silence the mutant ATXN3 *in vivo*, using a shRNA delivered by lentivirus targeting the **G/C** SNP. Lentiviral rat and mouse models, were generated through the stereotaxic injection of lentivirus in the striatum and in the cerebellum, respectively, allowing to evaluate neuropathological features before the onset of the symptoms. In these models, a significant improvement in the associated neuropathological deficits upon silencing of the mutant ATXN3 was observed, namely less intranuclear inclusions, preservation of neuronal markers, and less neurodegeneration [116, 117]. The study using the rat lentiviral model established the first proof-of-concept for allele-specific gene silencing in the central nervous system (CNS) [116]. The allele-specific gene silencing in the cerebellum of the lentiviral mouse model also prevented the appearance of balance and motor coordination abnormalities and reduced the hyperactivity in the animals [117]. Additionally, in a severely impaired transgenic mouse model, especially useful for an evaluation after the disease onset, it was observed a rescue of the disease-associated motor disabilities and mitigation of the neuropathological deficits [118]. Moreover, considering the numerous reports of cytotoxic effects associated with the RNAi technology, the safety profile of the previously developed and tested shRNA, delivered by a lentivirus, was assessed. Upon brain injection, the stable and long-term expression of the shRNA in the striatum of wild-type mice did not lead to toxic effects. Indeed, no abnormal neuronal dysfunction, astrocytic activation, microglial activity and proinflammatory cytokines release, off-target effects or saturation of the endogenous RNAi processing machinery was detected five months after the injection of the lentiviral vectors. Similar results were obtained in human cell cultures for potential off-target effects and saturation of the endogenous RNAi processing machinery. This well-structured and complete study constitutes an important step in a future translation of gene silencing as therapy for MJD/SCA3 [136].

In a less invasive approach, following the validation of its efficacy in neuronal cells, an exo-siRNA, encapsulated in SNALPs, targeting the **G/C** SNP was administered intravenously in two different mouse models of MJD/SCA3 (lentiviral and transgenic mouse models). The SNALPs had covalently attached to the surface a small peptide derived from rabies virus glycoprotein (RVG-9r) that confers brain-targeting capability (ability to cross the blood-brain barrier (BBB); -RVG counterpart), as well as improves the cellular uptake and the cytosolic release (-9r, nine arginines counterpart). The administration of the exo-siRNA encapsulated in SNALPs resulted in a selective and efficient silencing of mutant ATXN3, a reduction of the neuropathological inclusions, and an improvement of the motor behavior deficits [119].

Differently, and in a **G/C** SNP-independent manner, some allele-specific approaches have been focused on the CAG repeat expansion. Several mismatch-containing exo-siRNAs delivered by a liposome-based vector and targeting the CAG repeat expansion successfully decreased the mutant ATXN3 protein levels, in MJD/SCA3 patient-derived fibroblasts, with minor effects on the wild-type ATXN3 levels [120]. Another study, also targeting the CAG repeat expansion, tried to develop an allele-specific approach for four polyQ diseases — MJD/SCA3, SCA7, HD, and DRPLA. The strategy demonstrated the efficacy and allele selectivity of a shRNA delivered by lentivirus in the silencing of all four mutant proteins, including the mutant ATXN3, using patient-derived fibroblasts. Additionally, an evaluation of potential off-target effects revealed that the shRNA does not induce a significant degradation of other complementary transcripts [121].

An alternative approach reported a potent and allele-selective inhibition of the mutant ATXN3 expression using chemically modified single-stranded exo-siRNAs (ss-exo-siRNAs) targeting the CAG repeat expansion, in MJD/SCA3 patient-derived fibroblasts. It was also observed that the ss-exo-siRNAs, which were delivered by a liposome-based vector, bind to argonaute (argonaute-2) and promote its recruitment to the ATXN3 mRNA, validating the involvement of the RNAi pathway in the gene silencing mediated by ss-exo-siRNAs. Besides the RNAi mechanism, a non-RNAi-related process was found to affect the gene expression after the addition of the ss-exo-siRNAs, the alternative splicing, which is a typical mode of action of the antisense oligonucleotides (ASOs). Altogether, this approach shows that chemically modified ss-exo-siRNAs have properties of conventional exo-siRNAs and ASOs. Like exo-siRNAs, the ss-exo-siRNAs can operate through the RNAi pathway, and like ASOs, the ss-exo-siRNAs are single-stranded, simplifying their synthesis and chemical modification, and can trigger the alternative splicing [122].

2.2 Artificial microRNA and microRNA mimic-mediated gene silencing

As previously mentioned, an artificial miRNA consists of an exo-siRNA and a scaffold based on a natural pri-miRNA [97]. Considering that, similarly to exo-siRNAs, the gene silencing mediated by artificial miRNAs can be divided into non-allele-specific or allele-specific gene silencing. In a non-allele-specific approach, an artificial miRNA targeting the 3′ UTR of ATXN3 mRNA and delivered by adeno-associated virus (AAVs) was able to decrease efficiently the human mutant ATXN3 expression in the cerebellum of a transgenic mouse model of MJD/SCA3 [123, 124]. It was also observed less neuronal nuclear accumulation of the mutant ATXN3. In addition, the silencing of the mutant ATXN3 resulted in a partial normalization of the endogenous miRNA steady-state levels in mice. Although the mouse wild-type ATXN3 expression has not been affected *in vivo*, the artificial miRNA led to a significant reduction of the human wild-type ATXN3 expression in human cell cultures [123]. Furthermore, the administration of the artificial miRNA encoded by AAVs was not neurotoxic and did not lead to signs of astrogliosis or microgliosis [124]. In another non-allele-specific gene silencing approach, artificial miRNAs were engineered to target several exons within the ATXN3 mRNA. Based on their silencing efficacy in cell cultures, the three most promising candidates encoded by AAVs were further tested in human induced pluripotent stem cell (iPSC)-derived neurons and in a heterozygous knock-in mouse model of MJD/SCA3. It was observed an efficient reduction of the mutant ATXN3 expression, as well as a reduction of the wild-type ATXN3 expression, *in vivo* and *in vitro*, respectively. No evidence for off-target effects or saturation of the endogenous RNAi processing machinery was found in human iPSC-derived neurons. In addition, the authors demonstrated in a large mammal, the minipig, that an intrathecal administration of AAVs (AAV serotype 5) can simultaneously transduce the cerebellum and brain stem, the main areas affected in MJD/SCA3 patients [125].

Some miRNA screening studies on MJD/SCA3 have shown that the expression of several miRNAs is dysregulated and closely associated with the neuropathology in SCA3/MJD [137, 138]. Since the miRNA mimics are generated to behave as endogenous miRNAs, and its guide strand is designed to correspond to a naturally occurring mature miRNA, the miRNA mimics are particularly useful to restore the function of a miRNA downregulated in a disease condition [98, 99]. That was accomplished on MJD/SCA3 using miR-25, which was found to be significantly downregulated in the serum of patients. Following transfection, the upregulation of miR-25 strongly reduced both the mutant ATXN3 and wild-type ATXN3 levels, by interacting with the 3′ UTR of the mRNA, in human cell cultures. miR-25 also decreased protein aggregation, suppressed early apoptosis, and increased cell viability [126]. A different study identified three miRNAs — mir-9, mir-181a, and mir-494 — whose expression is downregulated in human MJD/SCA3 iPSC-derived neurons and other MJD/SCA3 cellular and animal models. All of them interact with the 3′ UTR of the mRNA and are highly expressed in the brain. The reestablishment of the three miRNAs, encoded by plasmids or lentivirus, led to an efficient reduction of human mutant ATXN3 levels in human cell cultures and a lentiviral mouse model, and a decrease of the protein aggregation and neuronal dysfunction in the lentiviral mouse model. The upregulation of mir-9 and mir-181a also affected the mouse wild-type ATXN3 levels *in vivo*. Additionally, the authors verified that the absence of the 3' UTR of the ATXN3, as a binding site for endogenous miRNAs, and the genetic and pharmacologic blockage of the miRNA biogenesis exacerbate the pathologic features of MJD/SCA3, *in vitro* and/or *in vivo* [127].

Another interesting but different study, based on a miRNA overexpression but not using miRNA mimics, performing an enhancer-promoter (EP) screen for modifiers through overexpression, showed that the miRNA bantam is a potent modulator in the neuropathology of MJD/SCA3 in a *Drosophila* model. The upregulation of the miRNA bantam suppressed the degenerative eye phenotype induced by the mutant ATXN3 toxicity. Surprisingly, miRNA bantam had no effect on the mutant ATXN3 protein levels. It was also verified that compromising the miRNA pathway/miRNA processing dramatically enhances the degeneration in the eyes of the *Drosophila* model and cell death in a human cell model of MJD/SCA3 [139]. Even though the miRNA bantam is not conserved between *Drosophila* and mammals, this study, together with the previous ones, suggests that the miRNA pathway/miRNAs have an important role in the neuropathology of MJD/SCA3.

3. Conclusions

An enormous effort was made by researchers to develop several gene silencing strategies based on RNAi molecules for MJD/SCA3. The results obtained decisively point to a huge therapeutic potential of these molecules. Overall, most of the studies showed both using allele or non-allele-specific strategies that various pathological features are mitigated, including in rodent models. Additionally, in several of these studies, the safety profile of the RNAi molecules was also assessed, corroborating their safety and increasing their therapeutic value. Nevertheless, an additional effort must be made to translate these preclinical results to human clinics, starting with their testing in clinical trials (searching on clinicalstrials.gov, there are no RNAi-based clinical trials yet). The approval in Europe and the US of an RNAi-based gene therapy for hereditary amyloid transthyretin (hATTR) amyloidosis, ONPATTRO® (patisiran), opens the way for these therapies and provides new hope for the RNAi-based gene therapies for MJD/SCA3 and other polyglutamine diseases.

Acknowledgements

We want to thank the projects and institutions funding Clévio Nóbrega laboratory, including the Portuguese Science and Technology Foundation (FCT) project (ALG-01-0145-FEDER-29480), "SeGrPolyQ" with CRESC ALGARVE 2020 cofunding, the French Muscular Dystrophy Association (AFM-Téléthon), ATAXIA UK, and the CureCSB project. JMC is supported by a Ph.D. fellowship from FCT (SFRH/BD/148760/2019).

Conflict of interest

The authors declare no conflict of interest.

Author details

José M. Codêsso, Carlos A. Matos and Clévio Nóbrega*
Faculty of Medicine and Biomedical Sciences, Algarve Biomedical Center — Research Institute (ABC-RI), University of Algarve, Faro, Portugal

*Address all correspondence to: cdnobrega@ualg.pt

References

[1] Coutinho P, Andrade C. Autosomal dominant system degeneration in Portuguese families of the Azores Islands. A new genetic disorder involving cerebellar, pyramidal, extrapyramidal and spinal cord motor functions. Neurology. 1978;**28**:703-709

[2] Rosenberg RN. Machado-Joseph disease: An autosomal dominant motor system degeneration. Movement Disorders. 1992;**7**:193-203

[3] Ranum LP, Lundgren JK, Schut LJ, Ahrens MJ, Perlman S, Aita J, et al. Spinocerebellar ataxia type 1 and Machado-Joseph disease: Incidence of CAG expansions among adult-onset ataxia patients from 311 families with dominant, recessive, or sporadic ataxia. American Journal of Human Genetics. 1995;**57**:603-608

[4] Schols L, Bauer P, Schmidt T, Schulte T, Riess O. Autosomal dominant cerebellar ataxias: Clinical features, genetics, and pathogenesis. Lancet Neurology. 2004;**3**:291-304

[5] Jardim LB, Silveira I, Pereira ML, Ferro A, Alonso I, et al. A survey of spinocerebellar ataxia in South Brazil - 66 new cases with Machado-Joseph disease, SCA7, SCA8, or unidentified disease-causing mutations. Journal of Neurology. 2001;**248**:870-876

[6] Silveira I, Coutinho P, Maciel P, Gaspar C, Hayes S, Dias A, et al. Analysis of SCA1, DRPLA, MJD, SCA2, and SCA6 CAG repeats in 48 Portuguese ataxia families. American Journal of Medical Genetics. 1998;**81**:134-138

[7] Vale J, Bugalho P, Silveira I, Sequeiros J, Guimaraes J, Coutinho P. Autosomal dominant cerebellar ataxia: Frequency analysis and clinical characterization of 45 families from Portugal. European Journal of Neurology. 2010;**17**:124-128

[8] Tang B, Liu C, Shen L, Dai H, Pan Q, Jing L, et al. Frequency of SCA1, SCA2, SCA3/MJD, SCA6, SCA7, and DRPLA CAG trinucleotide repeat expansion in patients with hereditary spinocerebellar ataxia from Chinese kindreds. Archives of Neurology. 2000;**57**:540-544

[9] Schols L, Amoiridis G, Buttner T, Przuntek H, Epplen JT, Riess O. Autosomal dominant cerebellar ataxia: Phenotypic differences in genetically defined subtypes? Annals of Neurology. 1997;**42**:924-932

[10] Maruyama H, Izumi Y, Morino H, Oda M, Toji H, Nakamura S, et al. Difference in disease-free survival curve and regional distribution according to subtype of spinocerebellar ataxia: A study of 1,286 Japanese patients. American Journal of Medical Genetics. 2002;**114**:578-583

[11] Shibata-Hamaguchi A, Ishida C, Iwasa K, Yamada M. Prevalence of spinocerebellar degenerations in the Hokuriku district in Japan. Neuroepidemiology. 2009;**32**:176-183

[12] Sudarsky L, Coutinho P. Machado-Joseph disease. Clinical Neuroscience. 1995;**3**:17-22

[13] Taroni F, DiDonato S. Pathways to motor incoordination: The inherited ataxias. Nature Reviews. Neuroscience. 2004;**5**:641-655

[14] Lima L, Coutinho P. Clinical criteria for diagnosis of Machado-Joseph disease: Report of a non-Azorena Portuguese family. Neurology. 1980;**30**:319-322

[15] Sequeiros J, Coutinho P. Epidemiology and clinical aspects of Machado-Joseph disease. Advances in Neurology. 1993;**61**:139-153

[16] D'Abreu A, Franca MC Jr, Paulson HL, Lopes-Cendes I. Caring for Machado-Joseph disease: Current understanding and how to help patients. Parkinsonism & Related Disorders. 2010;**16**:2-7

[17] Bettencourt C, Lima M. Machado-Joseph Disease: From first descriptions to new perspectives. Orphanet Journal of Rare Diseases. 2011;**6**:35

[18] Mendonca N, Franca MC Jr, Goncalves AF, Januario C. Clinical Features of Machado-Joseph Disease. Advances in Experimental Medicine and Biology. 2018;**1049**:255-273

[19] Rub U, Brunt ER, Deller T. New insights into the pathoanatomy of spinocerebellar ataxia type 3 (Machado-Joseph disease). Current Opinion in Neurology. 2008;**21**:111-116

[20] Scherzed W, Brunt ER, Heinsen H, de Vos RA, Seidel K, Burk K, et al. Pathoanatomy of cerebellar degeneration in spinocerebellar ataxia type 2 (SCA2) and type 3 (SCA3). Cerebellum. 2012;**11**:749-760

[21] Kawaguchi Y, Okamoto T, Taniwaki M, Aizawa M, Inoue M, Katayama S, et al. CAG expansions in a novel gene for Machado-Joseph disease at chromosome 14q32.1. Nature Genetics. 1994;**8**:221-228

[22] Cummings CJ, Zoghbi HY. Trinucleotide repeats: Mechanisms and pathophysiology. Annual Review of Genomics and Human Genetics. 2000;**1**:281-328

[23] Maciel P, Costa MC, Ferro A, Rousseau M, Santos CS, Gaspar C, et al. Improvement in the molecular diagnosis of Machado-Joseph disease. Archives of Neurology. 2001;**58**:1821-1827

[24] Maciel P, Gaspar C, DeStefano AL, Silveira I, Coutinho P, Radvany J, et al. Correlation between CAG repeat length and clinical features in Machado-Joseph disease. American Journal of Human Genetics. 1995;**57**:54-61

[25] Durcan TM, Kontogiannea M, Thorarinsdottir T, Fallon L, Williams AJ, Djarmati A, et al. The Machado-Joseph disease-associated mutant form of ataxin-3 regulates parkin ubiquitination and stability. Human Molecular Genetics. 2011;**20**:141-154

[26] Wang H, Ying Z, Wang G. Ataxin-3 regulates aggresome formation of copper-zinc superoxide dismutase (SOD1) by editing K63-linked polyubiquitin chains. The Journal of Biological Chemistry. 2012;**287**:28576-28585

[27] Li F, Macfarlan T, Pittman RN, Chakravarti D. Ataxin-3 is a histone-binding protein with two independent transcriptional corepressor activities. The Journal of Biological Chemistry. 2002;**277**:45004-45012

[28] Evert BO, Araujo J, Vieira-Saecker AM, de Vos RA, Harendza S, Klockgether T, et al. Ataxin-3 represses transcription via chromatin binding, interaction with histone deacetylase 3, and histone deacetylation. The Journal of Neuroscience. 2006;**26**:11474-11486

[29] Chatterjee A, Saha S, Chakraborty A, Silva-Fernandes A, Mandal SM, Neves-Carvalho A, et al. The role of the mammalian DNA end-processing enzyme polynucleotide kinase 3'-phosphatase in spinocerebellar ataxia type 3 pathogenesis. PLoS Genetics. 2015;**11**:e1004749

[30] Pfeiffer A, Luijsterburg MS, Acs K, Wiegant WW, Helfricht A, Herzog LK, et al. Ataxin-3 consolidates the MDC1-dependent DNA double-strand break response by counteracting the SUMO-targeted ubiquitin ligase RNF4. The EMBO Journal. 2017;**36**:1066-1083

[31] Paulson HL, Perez MK, Trottier Y, Trojanowski JQ, Subramony SH, Das SS, et al. Intranuclear inclusions of expanded polyglutamine protein in spinocerebellar ataxia type 3. Neuron. 1997;**19**:333-344

[32] Rub U, Brunt ER, Petrasch-Parwez E, Schols L, Theegarten D, Auburger G, et al. Degeneration of ingestion-related brainstem nuclei in spinocerebellar ataxia type 2, 3, 6 and 7. Neuropathology and Applied Neurobiology. 2006;**32**:635-649

[33] Schmidt T, Landwehrmeyer GB, Schmitt I, Trottier Y, Auburger G, Laccone F, et al. An isoform of ataxin-3 accumulates in the nucleus of neuronal cells in affected brain regions of SCA3 patients. Brain Pathology. 1998;**8**:669-679

[34] Matos CA, de Almeida LP, Nobrega C. Machado-Joseph disease/spinocerebellar ataxia type 3: Lessons from disease pathogenesis and clues into therapy. Journal of Neurochemistry. 2019;**148**:8-28

[35] van der Krol AR, Mur LA, Beld M, Mol JN, Stuitje AR. Flavonoid genes in petunia: Addition of a limited number of gene copies may lead to a suppression of gene expression. The Plant Cell. 1990;**2**:291-299

[36] Napoli C, Lemieux C, Jorgensen R. Introduction of a chimeric chalcone synthase gene into petunia results in reversible co-suppression of homologous genes in trans. The Plant Cell. 1990;**2**:279-289

[37] Fire A, Xu S, Montgomery MK, Kostas SA, Driver SE, Mello CC. Potent and specific genetic interference by double-stranded RNA in Caenorhabditis elegans. Nature. 1998;**391**:806-811

[38] Hannon GJ. RNA interference. Nature. 2002;**418**:244-251

[39] Wang X, Wang P, Sun S, Darwiche S, Idnurm A, Heitman J. Transgene induced co-suppression during vegetative growth in Cryptococcus neoformans. PLoS Genetics. 2012;**8**:e1002885

[40] He L, Hannon GJ. MicroRNAs: Small RNAs with a big role in gene regulation. Nature Reviews. Genetics. 2004;**5**:522-531

[41] Siomi MC, Sato K, Pezic D, Aravin AA. PIWI-interacting small RNAs: The vanguard of genome defence. Nature Reviews. Molecular Cell Biology. 2011;**12**:246-258

[42] Piatek MJ, Werner A. Endogenous siRNAs: Regulators of internal affairs. Biochemical Society Transactions. 2014;**42**:1174-1179

[43] Bartel DP. MicroRNAs: Genomics, biogenesis, mechanism, and function. Cell. 2004;**116**:281-297

[44] Jones-Rhoades MW, Bartel DP, Bartel B. MicroRNAS and their regulatory roles in plants. Annual Review of Plant Biology. 2006;**57**:19-53

[45] Obbard DJ, Gordon KH, Buck AH, Jiggins FM. The evolution of RNAi as a defence against viruses and transposable elements. Philosophical Transactions of the Royal Society of London. Series B, Biological Sciences. 2009;**364**:99-115

[46] Svoboda P. Renaissance of mammalian endogenous RNAi. FEBS Letters. 2014;**588**:2550-2556

[47] Lee Y, Kim M, Han J, Yeom KH, Lee S, Baek SH, et al. MicroRNA genes are transcribed by RNA polymerase II. The EMBO Journal. 2004;**23**:4051-4060

[48] Cai X, Hagedorn CH, Cullen BR. Human microRNAs are processed from capped, polyadenylated transcripts that can also function as mRNAs. RNA. 2004;**10**:1957-1966

[49] Lee Y, Ahn C, Han J, Choi H, Kim J, Yim J, et al. The nuclear RNase III Drosha initiates microRNA processing. Nature. 2003;**425**:415-419

[50] Landthaler M, Yalcin A, Tuschl T. The human DiGeorge syndrome critical region gene 8 and Its D. melanogaster homolog are required for miRNA biogenesis. Current Biology. 2004;**14**:2162-2167

[51] Han J, Lee Y, Yeom KH, Kim YK, Jin H, Kim VN. The Drosha-DGCR8 complex in primary microRNA processing. Genes & Development. 2004;**18**:3016-3027

[52] Gregory RI, Yan KP, Amuthan G, Chendrimada T, Doratotaj B, Cooch N, et al. The Microprocessor complex mediates the genesis of microRNAs. Nature. 2004;**432**:235-240

[53] Kwon SC, Jang H, Shen S, Baek SC, Kim K, Yang J, et al. ERH facilitates microRNA maturation through the interaction with the N-terminus of DGCR8. Nucleic Acids Research. 2020;**48**:11097-11112

[54] Yi R, Qin Y, Macara IG, Cullen BR. Exportin-5 mediates the nuclear export of pre-microRNAs and short hairpin RNAs. Genes & Development. 2003;**17**:3011-3016

[55] Bohnsack MT, Czaplinski K, Gorlich D. Exportin 5 is a RanGTP-dependent dsRNA-binding protein that mediates nuclear export of pre-miRNAs. RNA. 2004;**10**:185-191

[56] Hutvagner G, McLachlan J, Pasquinelli AE, Balint E, Tuschl T, Zamore PD. A cellular function for the RNA-interference enzyme Dicer in the maturation of the let-7 small temporal RNA. Science. 2001;**293**:834-838

[57] Ketting RF, Fischer SE, Bernstein E, Sijen T, Hannon GJ, Plasterk RH. Dicer functions in RNA interference and in synthesis of small RNA involved in developmental timing in C. elegans. Genes & Development. 2001;**15**:2654-2659

[58] Haase AD, Jaskiewicz L, Zhang H, Laine S, Sack R, Gatignol A, et al. TRBP, a regulator of cellular PKR and HIV-1 virus expression, interacts with Dicer and functions in RNA silencing. EMBO Reports. 2005;**6**:961-967

[59] Lee Y, Hur I, Park SY, Kim YK, Suh MR, Kim VN. The role of PACT in the RNA silencing pathway. The EMBO Journal. 2006;**25**:522-532

[60] Chendrimada TP, Gregory RI, Kumaraswamy E, Norman J, Cooch N, Nishikura K, et al. TRBP recruits the Dicer complex to Ago2 for microRNA processing and gene silencing. Nature. 2005;**436**:740-744

[61] Gregory RI, Chendrimada TP, Cooch N, Shiekhattar R. Human RISC couples microRNA biogenesis and posttranscriptional gene silencing. Cell. 2005;**123**:631-640

[62] Janowski BA, Huffman KE, Schwartz JC, Ram R, Nordsell R, Shames DS, et al. Involvement of AGO1 and AGO2 in mammalian transcriptional silencing. Nature Structural & Molecular Biology. 2006;**13**:787-792

[63] Tabara H, Yigit E, Siomi H, Mello CC. The dsRNA binding protein RDE-4 interacts with RDE-1, DCR-1, and a DExH-box helicase to direct RNAi in C. elegans. Cell. 2002;**109**:861-871

[64] Robb GB, Rana TM. RNA helicase A interacts with RISC in human cells and functions in RISC loading. Molecular Cell. 2007;**26**:523-537

[65] Wang B, Li S, Qi HH, Chowdhury D, Shi Y, Novina CD. Distinct passenger strand and mRNA cleavage activities of human Argonaute proteins. Nature Structural & Molecular Biology. 2009;**16**:1259-1266

[66] Schwarz DS, Hutvagner G, Du T, Xu Z, Aronin N, Zamore PD. Asymmetry in the assembly of the RNAi enzyme complex. Cell. 2003;**115**:199-208

[67] Lewis BP, Shih IH, Jones-Rhoades MW, Bartel DP, Burge CB. Prediction of mammalian microRNA targets. Cell. 2003;**115**:787-798

[68] Lewis BP, Burge CB, Bartel DP. Conserved seed pairing, often flanked by adenosines, indicates that thousands of human genes are microRNA targets. Cell. 2005;**120**:15-20

[69] Grimson A, Farh KK, Johnston WK, Garrett-Engele P, Lim LP, Bartel DP. MicroRNA targeting specificity in mammals: Determinants beyond seed pairing. Molecular Cell. 2007;**27**:91-105

[70] Sheu-Gruttadauria J, Xiao Y, Gebert LF, MacRae IJ. Beyond the seed: Structural basis for supplementary microRNA targeting by human Argonaute2. The EMBO Journal. 2019;**38**:e101153

[71] Saxena S, Jonsson ZO, Dutta A. Small RNAs with imperfect match to endogenous mRNA repress translation. Implications for off-target activity of small inhibitory RNA in mammalian cells. Journal of Biological Chemistry. 2003;**278**:44312-44319

[72] Liu J, Valencia-Sanchez MA, Hannon GJ, Parker R. MicroRNA-dependent localization of targeted mRNAs to mammalian P-bodies. Nature Cell Biology. 2005;**7**:719-723

[73] Watanabe T, Takeda A, Tsukiyama T, Mise K, Okuno T, Sasaki H, et al. Identification and characterization of two novel classes of small RNAs in the mouse germline: Retrotransposon-derived siRNAs in oocytes and germline small RNAs in testes. Genes & Development. 2006;**20**:1732-1743

[74] Yang N, Kazazian HH Jr. L1 retrotransposition is suppressed by endogenously encoded small interfering RNAs in human cultured cells. Nature Structural & Molecular Biology. 2006;**13**:763-771

[75] Okamura K, Balla S, Martin R, Liu N, Lai EC. Two distinct mechanisms generate endogenous siRNAs from bidirectional transcription in Drosophila melanogaster. Nature Structural & Molecular Biology. 2008;**15**:998

[76] Tam OH, Aravin AA, Stein P, Girard A, Murchison EP, Cheloufi S, et al. Pseudogene-derived small interfering RNAs regulate gene expression in mouse oocytes. Nature. 2008;**453**:534-538

[77] Okamura K, Chung WJ, Ruby JG, Guo H, Bartel DP, Lai EC. The Drosophila hairpin RNA pathway generates endogenous short interfering RNAs. Nature. 2008;**453**:803-806

[78] Chung WJ, Okamura K, Martin R, Lai EC. Endogenous RNA interference provides a somatic defense against Drosophila transposons. Current Biology. 2008;**18**:795-802

[79] Ghildiyal M, Seitz H, Horwich MD, Li C, Du T, Lee S, et al. Endogenous siRNAs derived from transposons and mRNAs in Drosophila somatic cells. Science. 2008;**320**:1077-1081

[80] Kawamura Y, Saito K, Kin T, Ono Y, Asai K, Sunohara T, et al. Drosophila endogenous small RNAs bind to Argonaute 2 in somatic cells. Nature. 2008;**453**:793-797

[81] Watanabe T, Totoki Y, Toyoda A, Kaneda M, Kuramochi-Miyagawa S, Obata Y, et al. Endogenous siRNAs from naturally formed dsRNAs regulate transcripts in mouse oocytes. Nature. 2008;**453**:539-543

[82] Gunawardane LS, Saito K, Nishida KM, Miyoshi K, Kawamura Y, Nagami T, et al. A slicer-mediated mechanism for repeat-associated siRNA 5' end formation in Drosophila. Science. 2007;**315**:1587-1590

[83] Brennecke J, Aravin AA, Stark A, Dus M, Kellis M, Sachidanandam R, et al. Discrete small RNA-generating loci as master regulators of transposon activity in Drosophila. Cell. 2007;**128**:1089-1103

[84] Watanabe T, Chuma S, Yamamoto Y, Kuramochi-Miyagawa S, Totoki Y, Toyoda A, et al. MITOPLD is a mitochondrial protein essential for nuage formation and piRNA biogenesis in the mouse germline. Developmental Cell. 2011;**20**:364-375

[85] Nishimasu H, Ishizu H, Saito K, Fukuhara S, Kamatani MK, Bonnefond L, et al. Structure and function of Zucchini endoribonuclease in piRNA biogenesis. Nature. 2012;**491**:284-287

[86] Aravin AA, Sachidanandam R, Bourc'his D, Schaefer C, Pezic D, Toth KF, et al. A piRNA pathway primed by individual transposons is linked to de novo DNA methylation in mice. Molecular Cell. 2008;**31**:785-799

[87] Reuter M, Berninger P, Chuma S, Shah H, Hosokawa M, Funaya C, et al. Miwi catalysis is required for piRNA amplification-independent LINE1 transposon silencing. Nature. 2011;**480**:264-267

[88] Keam SP, Young PE, McCorkindale AL, Dang TH, Clancy JL, Humphreys DT, et al. The human Piwi protein Hiwi2 associates with tRNA-derived piRNAs in somatic cells. Nucleic Acids Research. 2014;**42**:8984-8995

[89] Wang W, Han BW, Tipping C, Ge DT, Zhang Z, Weng Z, et al. Slicing and Binding by Ago3 or Aub Trigger Piwi-Bound piRNA Production by Distinct Mechanisms. Molecular Cell. 2015;**59**:819-830

[90] Li C, Vagin VV, Lee S, Xu J, Ma S, Xi H, et al. Collapse of germline piRNAs in the absence of Argonaute3 reveals somatic piRNAs in flies. Cell. 2009;**137**:509-521

[91] De Fazio S, Bartonicek N, Di Giacomo M, Abreu-Goodger C, Sankar A, Funaya C, et al. The endonuclease activity of Mili fuels piRNA amplification that silences LINE1 elements. Nature. 2011;**480**:259-263

[92] Balaratnam S, West N, Basu S. A piRNA utilizes HILI and HIWI2 mediated pathway to down-regulate ferritin heavy chain 1 mRNA in human somatic cells. Nucleic Acids Research. 2018;**46**:10635-10648

[93] Matos CA, Carmona V, Vijayakumar UG, Lopes S, Albuquerque P, Conceicao M, et al. Gene therapies for polyglutamine diseases. Advances in Experimental Medicine and Biology. 2018;**1049**:395-438

[94] Rettig GR, Behlke MA. Progress toward in vivo use of siRNAs-II. Molecular Therapy. 2012;**20**:483-512

[95] Wittrup A, Lieberman J. Knocking down disease: A progress report on siRNA therapeutics. Nature Reviews. Genetics. 2015;**16**:543-552

[96] Fellmann C, Lowe SW. Stable RNA interference rules for silencing. Nature Cell Biology. 2014;**16**:10-18

[97] Kotowska-Zimmer A, Pewinska M, Olejniczak M. Artificial miRNAs as therapeutic tools: Challenges and opportunities. Wiley Interdiscip Rev RNA. 2021;**12**:e1640

[98] Bader AG, Brown D, Winkler M. The promise of microRNA replacement therapy. Cancer Research. 2010;**70**:7027-7030

[99] Rupaimoole R, Slack FJ. MicroRNA therapeutics: Towards a new era for the management of cancer and other diseases. Nature Reviews. Drug Discovery. 2017;**16**:203-222

[100] Yin H, Kanasty RL, Eltoukhy AA, Vegas AJ, Dorkin JR, Anderson DG. Non-viral vectors for gene-based therapy. Nature Reviews. Genetics. 2014;**15**:541-555

[101] Grimm D, Streetz KL, Jopling CL, Storm TA, Pandey K, Davis CR, et al. Fatality in mice due to oversaturation of cellular microRNA/short hairpin RNA pathways. Nature. 2006;**441**:537-541

[102] Yi R, Doehle BP, Qin Y, Macara IG, Cullen BR. Overexpression of exportin 5 enhances RNA interference mediated by short hairpin RNAs and microRNAs. RNA. 2005;**11**:220-226

[103] Bridge AJ, Pebernard S, Ducraux A, Nicoulaz AL, Iggo R. Induction of an interferon response by RNAi vectors in mammalian cells. Nature Genetics. 2003;**34**:263-264

[104] Hornung V, Ellegast J, Kim S, Brzozka K, Jung A, Kato H, et al. 5'-Triphosphate RNA is the ligand for RIG-I. Science. 2006;**314**:994-997

[105] Birmingham A, Anderson EM, Reynolds A, Ilsley-Tyree D, Leake D, Fedorov Y, et al. 3' UTR seed matches, but not overall identity, are associated with RNAi off-targets. Nature Methods. 2006;**3**:199-204

[106] Jackson AL, Burchard J, Schelter J, Chau BN, Cleary M, Lim L, et al. Widespread siRNA "off-target" transcript silencing mediated by seed region sequence complementarity. RNA. 2006;**12**:1179-1187

[107] Bauer PO, Nukina N. The pathogenic mechanisms of polyglutamine diseases and current therapeutic strategies. Journal of Neurochemistry. 2009;**110**:1737-1765

[108] Nalavade R, Griesche N, Ryan DP, Hildebrand S, Krauss S. Mechanisms of RNA-induced toxicity in CAG repeat disorders. Cell Death & Disease. 2013;**4**:e752

[109] Li LB, Yu Z, Teng X, Bonini NM. RNA toxicity is a component of ataxin-3 degeneration in Drosophila. Nature. 2008;**453**:1107-1111

[110] Wang LC, Chen KY, Pan H, Wu CC, Chen PH, Liao YT, et al. Muscleblind participates in RNA toxicity of expanded CAG and CUG repeats in Caenorhabditis elegans. Cellular and Molecular Life Sciences. 2011;**68**:1255-1267

[111] Ramani B, Harris GM, Huang R, Seki T, Murphy GG, Costa Mdo C, et al. A knockin mouse model

of spinocerebellar ataxia type 3 exhibits prominent aggregate pathology and aberrant splicing of the disease gene transcript. Human Molecular Genetics. 2015;**24**:1211-1224

[112] Alves S, Nascimento-Ferreira I, Dufour N, Hassig R, Auregan G, Nobrega C, et al. Silencing ataxin-3 mitigates degeneration in a rat model of Machado-Joseph disease: No role for wild-type ataxin-3? Human Molecular Genetics. 2010;**19**:2380-2394

[113] Hu J, Matsui M, Gagnon KT, Schwartz JC, Gabillet S, Arar K, et al. Inhibiting expression of mutant huntingtin and Ataxin-3 by targeting expanded CAG repeat RNAs. Nature Biotechnology. 2009;**27**:478-484

[114] Miller VM, Xia H, Marrs GL, Gouvion CM, Lee G, Davidson BL, et al. Allele-specific silencing of dominant disease genes. Proceedings of the National Academy of Sciences of the United States of America. 2003;**100**:7195-7200

[115] Li Y, Yokota T, Matsumura R, Taira K, Mizusawa H. Sequence-dependent and independent inhibition specific for mutant ataxin-3 by small interfering RNA. Annals of Neurology. 2004;**56**:124-129

[116] Alves S, Nascimento-Ferreira I, Auregan G, Hassig R, Dufour N, Brouillet E, et al. Allele-specific RNA silencing of mutant ataxin-3 mediates neuroprotection in a rat model of Machado-Joseph disease. PLoS One. 2008;**3**:e3341

[117] Nobrega C, Nascimento-Ferreira I, Onofre I, Albuquerque D, Deglon N, de Almeida LP. RNA interference mitigates motor and neuropathological deficits in a cerebellar mouse model of Machado-Joseph disease. PLoS One. 2014;**9**:e100086

[118] Nobrega C, Nascimento-Ferreira I, Onofre I, Albuquerque D, Hirai H, Deglon N, et al. Silencing mutant ataxin-3 rescues motor deficits and neuropathology in Machado-Joseph disease transgenic mice. PLoS One. 2013;**8**:e52396

[119] Conceicao M, Mendonca L, Nobrega C, Gomes C, Costa P, Hirai H, et al. Intravenous administration of brain-targeted stable nucleic acid lipid particles alleviates Machado-Joseph disease neurological phenotype. Biomaterials. 2016;**82**:124-137

[120] Hu J, Gagnon KT, Liu J, Watts JK, Syeda-Nawaz J, Bennett CF, et al. Allele-selective inhibition of ataxin-3 (ATX3) expression by antisense oligomers and duplex RNAs. Biological Chemistry. 2011;**392**:315-325

[121] Kotowska-Zimmer A, Ostrovska Y, Olejniczak M. Universal RNAi triggers for the specific inhibition of mutant Huntingtin, Atrophin-1, Ataxin-3, and Ataxin-7 Expression. Molecular Therapy--Nucleic Acids. 2020;**19**:562-571

[122] Liu J, Yu D, Aiba Y, Pendergraff H, Swayze EE, Lima WF, et al. ss-siRNAs allele selectively inhibit ataxin-3 expression: Multiple mechanisms for an alternative gene silencing strategy. Nucleic Acids Research. 2013;**41**:9570-9583

[123] Rodriguez-Lebron E, Costa Mdo C, Luna-Cancalon K, Peron TM, Fischer S, Boudreau RL, et al. Silencing mutant ATXN3 expression resolves molecular phenotypes in SCA3 transgenic mice. Molecular Therapy. 2013;**21**:1909-1918

[124] Costa Mdo C, Luna-Cancalon K, Fischer S, Ashraf NS, Ouyang M, Dharia RM, et al. Toward RNAi therapy for the polyglutamine disease

Machado-Joseph disease. Molecular Therapy. 2013;**21**:1898-1908

[125] Martier R, Sogorb-Gonzalez M, Stricker-Shaver J, Hubener-Schmid J, Keskin S, Klima J, et al. Development of an AAV-based MicroRNA gene therapy to treat Machado-Joseph disease. Mol Ther Methods Clin Dev. 2019;**15**:343-358

[126] Huang F, Zhang L, Long Z, Chen Z, Hou X, Wang C, et al. miR-25 alleviates polyQ-mediated cytotoxicity by silencing ATXN3. FEBS Letters. 2014;**588**:4791-4798

[127] Carmona V, Cunha-Santos J, Onofre I, Simoes AT, Vijayakumar U, Davidson BL, et al. Unravelling endogenous MicroRNA system dysfunction as a new pathophysiological mechanism in Machado-Joseph disease. Molecular Therapy. 2017;**25**:1038-1055

[128] Rodriguez-Lebron E, Paulson HL. Allele-specific RNA interference for neurological disease. Gene Therapy. 2006;**13**:576-581

[129] Scholefield J, Wood MJ. Therapeutic gene silencing strategies for polyglutamine disorders. Trends in Genetics. 2010;**26**:29-38

[130] Schmitt I, Linden M, Khazneh H, Evert BO, Breuer P, Klockgether T, et al. Inactivation of the mouse Atxn3 (ataxin-3) gene increases protein ubiquitination. Biochemical and Biophysical Research Communications. 2007;**362**:734-739

[131] Rodrigues AJ, Coppola G, Santos C, Costa Mdo C, Ailion M, Sequeiros J, et al. Functional genomics and biochemical characterization of the C. elegans orthologue of the Machado-Joseph disease protein ataxin-3. The FASEB Journal. 2007;**21**:1126-1136

[132] Zeng L, Zhang D, McLoughlin HS, Zalon AJ, Aravind L, Paulson HL. Loss of the Spinocerebellar Ataxia type 3 disease protein ATXN3 alters transcription of multiple signal transduction pathways. PLoS One. 2018;**13**:e0204438

[133] Stevanin G, Cancel G, Didierjean O, Durr A, Abbas N, Cassa E, et al. Linkage disequilibrium at the Machado-Joseph disease/spinal cerebellar ataxia 3 locus: Evidence for a common founder effect in French and Portuguese-Brazilian families as well as a second ancestral Portuguese-Azorean mutation. American Journal of Human Genetics. 1995;**57**:1247-1250

[134] Gaspar C, Lopes-Cendes I, DeStefano AL, Maciel P, Silveira I, Coutinho P, et al. Linkage disequilibrium analysis in Machado-Joseph disease patients of different ethnic origins. Human Genetics. 1996;**98**:620-624

[135] Gaspar C, Lopes-Cendes I, Hayes S, Goto J, Arvidsson K, Dias A, et al. Ancestral origins of the Machado-Joseph disease mutation: A worldwide haplotype study. American Journal of Human Genetics. 2001;**68**:523-528

[136] Nobrega C, Codesso JM, Mendonca L, Pereira de Almeida L. RNA interference therapy for Machado-Joseph disease: Long-term safety profile of lentiviral vectors encoding short hairpin RNAs targeting mutant Ataxin-3. Human Gene Therapy. 2019;**30**:841-854

[137] Shi Y, Huang F, Tang B, Li J, Wang J, Shen L, et al. MicroRNA profiling in the serums of SCA3/MJD patients. The International Journal of Neuroscience. 2014;**124**:97-101

[138] Krauss S, Nalavade R, Weber S, Carter K, Evert BO. Upregulation of miR-25 and miR-181 family members correlates with reduced expression of

ATXN3 in lymphocytes from SCA3 patients. Microrna. 2019;**8**:76-85

[139] Bilen J, Liu N, Burnett BG, Pittman RN, Bonini NM. MicroRNA pathways modulate polyglutamine-induced neurodegeneration. Molecular Cell. 2006;**24**:157-163